Co-creating and Co-producing Research Evidence

The importance of a strong evidence-base is widely recognised in contemporary health, social care and education practice, meaning that there is a real need for research which can be quickly and easily translated into real world situations.

Research co-produced by practitioners and academics from early stages to end results can draw on each party's knowledge and experience, in order to create high quality evidence that is relevant and appropriate to practice needs. This guide introduces the basics of co-producing research, looking at the evidence for co-produced research and outlining its theoretical underpinnings, as well as discussing barriers and facilitators to consider. It includes a practitioner perspective and an academic perspective on the benefits and challenges of co-produced research. The substantive chapters are each co-written by an academic and practitioner team and give examples of work carried out – and lessons learned – in public health, education and criminal justice settings. Key learning points are included throughout and drawn together to comprise a toolkit at the end of the book.

This book teaches academics and practitioners more about how they can find practical evidence-based answers to complex questions.

Dorothy Newbury-Birch is Professor of Alcohol and Public Health Research at the School of Social Sciences, Humanities and Law at Teesside University where she leads a team of researchers and postgraduate students.

Keith Allan is a Consultant in Public Health. He has a Master's in Public Health Research, University of Edinburgh, and a PhD in Child Health, University of Aberdeen.

Co-creating and Co-producing Research Evidence

A Guide for Practitioners and Academics in Health, Social Care and Education Settings

Edited by
Dorothy Newbury-Birch and Keith Allan

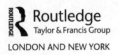

Routledge
Taylor & Francis Group

LONDON AND NEW YORK

First published 2020
by Routledge
2 Park Square, Milton Park, Abingdon, Oxon OX14 4RN

and by Routledge
52 Vanderbilt Avenue, New York, NY 10017

Routledge is an imprint of the Taylor & Francis Group, an informa business

British Library Cataloguing in Publication Data
A catalogue record for this book is available from the British Library

Library of Congress Cataloging-in-Publication Data
A catalog record has been requested for this book

ISBN: 978-1-138-57900-2 (hbk)
ISBN: 978-1-138-57901-9 (pbk)
ISBN: 978-1-351-26300-9 (ebk)

Typeset in Times New Roman
by Taylor & Francis Books
Printed by CPI Group (UK) Ltd, Croydon CR0 4YY

For Victor Birch and Ian Newbury who believed in me (Dorothy Newbury-Birch). To all those engaged in the co-production of health and wellbeing; to those who blur the lines between practitioner, researcher, professional and service user in the pursuit of salutogenesis (Keith Allan).

Contents

Illustrations

Figure

Tables

Box

Contributors

Dorothy Newbury-Birch is Professor of Alcohol and Public Health Research and the Director of the Centre for Crime, Harm Prevention and Security at the School of Social Sciences, Humanities and Law at Teesside University where she leads a team of researchers and postgraduate students. Her overarching research programme aims to reduce the risks and harms of alcohol in society. In particular, this is with two distinct groups: those in the criminal justice system, and young people. Her research is very much focussed on how we narrow the gap between academics, practitioners and service users in public health and within the criminal justice system. To date she have been a co-applicant on over £14 million in research grants from national and international sources. Of this, she has been the Chief Investigator on grants worth £1.6 million. She has been involved in nearly 100 publications including publications in The Lancet (lead author) and the BMJ, Addiction and Journal of Experimental Criminology (co-author) and has been named on numerous governmental reports around restorative justice and also around alcohol misuse. Dorothy lives in the North Yorkshire Moors with her ever-patient husband and four dogs.

Keith Allan is a consultant in public health. Twin interests in epidemiology and social justice prompted him to enter the field of public health through an MSc in Public Health Research at the University of Edinburgh. This led to a PhD in child health, working with the SEATON birth cohort, and post-doctoral work at the University of Aberdeen looking at the lifelong health impacts of maternal weight change in pregnancy to adult offspring. Subsequently moving to work in public health in the North East of England, Keith had the opportunity to participate in co-production and translational research with colleagues and wider stakeholders. As a consultant in public health in Scotland, Keith continues to use evidence-based practice to support the health of the population and maintains a keen interest in delivering meaningful co-produced change to improve the health of individuals and the community. Keith lives in the Scottish countryside with his fiancée and their two cats.

Michelle Baldwin is a Public Health Strategic Manager, Durham County Council.

Daniel Barber is a former pupil at Norham High School, North Tyneside.

Jane Bourne is a drama therapist in the Arts Therapies Team, Northumberland, Tyne and Wear NHS Foundation Trust.

Scott Brown is a former pupil at Norham High School, North Tyneside.

Michael Chay-Hayden is a former pupil at Norham High School, North Tyneside.

Mandy Cheetham is a post-doctoral research associate in the School of Health and Social Care at Teesside University and currently works as an embedded researcher with the Public Health team at Gateshead Council.

Natalie Connor is a post-doctoral research associate in the School of Social Sciences, Humanities and Law at Teesside University, working on coproduction evaluations with the Public Health team at Durham County Council.

Paul Croney is Vice Chancellor and Chief Executive at Teesside University.

Louisa J. Ells is Professor of Public Health and Obesity at the School of Health and Social Care at Teesside University and holds a part time secondment as specialist academic advisor to public Health England.

Jennifer Ferguson is a graduate tutor and PhD student at Teesside University.

Emma Gibson is a Public Health Programme Lead at Gateshead Council.

Emma L. Giles is a reader in Public Health and Behaviour Change in the School of Health and Social Care at Teesside University.

Sarah Gorman is chief executive of Edberts House in Gateshead.

Victoria Guthrie is a senior research fellow at the School of Health in Social Sciences at the University of Edinburgh.

Sean Harris is the North of England area director for Ambition School Leadership and former Deputy Headteacher at Norham High School.

Mark Hatcher is a former police officer, Northumbria Police.

Abbey Hodgson is a former pupil at Norham High School, North Tyneside.

Aisha Holloway is Professor of Nursing Studies and Head of Nursing Studies at the School of Health in Social Sciences at the University of Edinburgh.

Lewis Hudson is a former pupil at Norham High School, North Tyneside. C/O

Grant J. McGeechan is a senior lecturer in Health Psychology in the School of Social Sciences, Humanities and Law, Teesside University

Katie Miller is a former pupil at Norham High School, North Tyneside.

Gill O'Neill is the Deputy Director of Public Health within Durham County Council.

Tony Power, former police officer, Northumbria Police and current law student at Canterbury Christ Church University.

Joan Roberts, manager, School Health Research Network (SHRN), DECIPHer Centre, Cardiff University.

Jeremy Segrott is a lecturer in the Centre for Trials Research and DECIPHer Centre at Cardiff University, Wales, UK.

Claire Sullivan is the Deputy Director Health, Wellbeing and Workforce at Public Health England.

Angela Tomlinson is a police constable with Northumbria Police Force.

Mick Urwin is a Sergeant with Durham Police Force.

Gillian Waller is a post-doctoral research associate in the School of Social Sciences, Humanities and Law at Teesside University.

Kirsty Wilkinson is a Public Health Advanced Practitioner at Durham County Council.

Alice Wiseman is Director of Public Health at Gateshead Council.

Dianne Woodall is a Public Health Portfolio Lead at Durham County Council.

Foreword

I am delighted to be asked to write the foreword to this book *Co-creating and Co-producing Research Evidence: A Guide for Practitioners and Academics in Health, Social Care and Education Settings*, which is co-edited by Professor Dorothy Newbury-Birch from the School of Social Sciences, Humanities and Law at Teesside University and Dr Keith Allan who is a Consultant in Public Health in Melrose, Scotland and published by Routledge.

Teesside is a leading university with an international reputation for academic excellence that provides an outstanding student and learning experience underpinned by research, enterprise and the professions. One of the strategic aims of the university is to carry out world-leading and internationally excellent research than informs learning and teaching, partner activity and knowledge transfer. One of the ways that we are doing this is in supporting an interdisciplinary solution to address key global societal challenges of our time through our Grand Challenge Research Themes: health and wellbeing; resilient and secure societies; digital and creative economy; sustainable environments and learning for the twenty-first century.

This new and innovative book will help academics and practitioners to work together more effectively to deliver research findings that have a direct influence on individuals lives. I am particularly impressed with the range of work highlighted in the book including work in schools (Chapters 4 and 5), the criminal justice system (Chapters 9 and 10) and public health teams (Chapters 6, 7 and 8). Chapter 5 is co-written with young people from Norham High School in the North East of England who have worked with Professor Newbury-Birch on a piece of co-production research around the effect of the new GCSEs on staff and students. The young people developed, carried out the research and wrote up the results with the academic team from here at Teesside. It is work like this that will help develop the next generation of researchers.

Professor Paul Croney,
Vice Chancellor and Chief Executive,
Teesside University

1   Why should we co-produce research?

Claire Sullivan and Gill O'Neill

Understanding the context

Understanding the context a co-production project is to be conducted in is key and can include prioritising limited resources to meet health needs, something of a particular challenge in areas like the North East of England where health outcomes remain stubbornly lower than the England average and where there is substantial (perceived or actual) unmet heath needs. There is much to consider with regard to how interventions are evaluated to demonstrate adding value to the local system without the requirement for a randomised control trial.

There is prolific delivery in local public health teams where the evidence base has been interpreted and applied within the local context but we are often left unsure of whether there is a difference being made to local people/ recipients of the interventions unless robust evaluation is wrapped around an intervention.

Additionally, there is perhaps an assumption that commissioning decisions are linear. These decisions are subject to strict funding regimes, are bound in political tensions (national and local), follow a strict timeline and are led by one individual whose focus is just on that commission.

Considering all of the above, the importance of the context is clear. Good understanding of its potential impact by researchers is therefore clearly beneficial and can be supported through the co-production process. This is likely to provide deeper learning and robust research findings that are more likely to be applicable to the environment a practitioner works within.

Translational research and translational practice

Having worked in public health practice for some time, we have also advocated that the focus on 'translational research' or knowledge exchange, has often been considered as one directional – how to get the research evidence into practice. There is often a very long time lag to get published research into practice with this taking as long as 17 years (Morris et al. 2011). Yet rarely do we hear how can practice inform research. The more recent focus on the need for research funders to look at 'natural experiments' is promising but under-utilised (Petticrew et al. 2005).

Case studies are used to share 'good' or 'promising' practice – but who said it's good and will it translate here? Therefore, case studies are read with interest but are often not replicated as the local context remains pivotal to successful implementation.

Implementation science is commonly defined as the study of methods and strategies to promote the uptake of interventions that have proven effective into routine practice, with the aim of improving population health. Implementation science therefore examines what works, for whom and under what circumstances, and how interventions can be adapted and scaled up in ways that are accessible and equitable (Michie et al. 2009). The field of implementation science has been born as a result of recognising the importance of the gap between research and practice (Glasgow et al. 2003). This gap has expedited the use of multitudinous theoretical constructs, aiming to enhance the implementation process, identify the barriers and facilitators and acting as valuable tools in evaluating implementation (May and Finch 2009). For public health practitioners endeavouring to implement evidence based practice, understanding the barriers and enablers to practical implementation are critical in the field. Undertaking local level evaluation, with implementation science domains, is a step towards understanding the context in which to apply evidence based research.

Academic drivers

One of the major barriers to engaging academics in co-production work within certain public health practitioner settings is the constraint put on the type of experiment that can be conducted. It would be unusual to be able to carry out a randomised controlled trial (RCT) in a local authority setting for example. While some methods would allow controlled evaluation of new initiatives as they are rolled out (e.g. stepped wedge cluster randomised trial) (Hemming et al. 2015), the majority of projects are likely to be observational or implementation studies. Due to the hierarchy of evidence and the academic drive to publish in high impact journals these settings may initially seem less attractive to academics (Newbury-Birch et al. 2016). However, through engaging in such co-production projects academics will gain access to new types of data and study subjects and may, for example, provide an excellent opportunity to generate important qualitative research (Newbury-Birch et al. 2016). Furthermore, it provides a welcome opportunity for academics to see their research put into practice. In order to create robust partnerships these benefits should be strongly communicated.

How did the co-production journey begin?

Research is expensive

Whilst working at a former Primary Care Trust, we were keen to understand the emotional and financial impact for patients and their families living with cancer. The 'intervention' was the provision of dedicated welfare rights support officers in the County to provide the advice during this difficult time for individuals and their families. We were keen to evaluate the impact of such a scheme, yet the research was going to cost twice that of the intervention due to the full economic cost (FEC) applied by academic institutions. A cost simply unpalatable to Local Government colleagues. The solution in the end was to use a third party – a charity where the FEC did not apply. At the same time some commissioners were engaging independent contractors to help with some process evaluations at the cost of approximately ten thousand pounds each using underspend funding. Some of these evaluations were poor in quality and lacked the methodological rigour as they were not being led by academic institutions. The risk with this is that glossy published reports are produced that look impressive to commissioners but have substantial flaws in their recommendations and thus renders them less than useful.

So, what was the model?

As a result of the difficulties and barriers described above, we agreed it would be more effective and cost effective to employ a researcher for a year rather than spend the small sums of funding on poor quality discrete pieces. The postholder was employed by a university, worked for three days a week in the Institute and two days a week in the practice location. Thus, the embedded researcher became straddled across two worlds – the researcher in the middle then benefitted from understanding the context of place, priorities and politics (Newbury-Birch et al. 2016).

A steering group was established to agree the areas of practice that would benefit from rapid evaluations, and the practitioners leading these workstreams became aligned with the researcher to drive forward the research programmes.

What are the benefits?

Increasing research capacity of practitioners

To ensure the embedded researcher wasn't simply just undertaking academic traditional research but from a different office base, the public health practitioners leading on the areas of work being evaluated were given the opportunity to work alongside the researcher and a co-production model was created.

To enable this co-production model to be developed there were some practical barriers to overcome such as the majority of PH practitioners not having access to a university Athens account and therefore not having access to up-to-date evidence and journals. The model applied in County Durham, at a time when Athens was not available to the practitioners, was to ensure they had access to the university library and could also step outside their world and institute into another. This step to improve access to evidence, to be able to critically review it using a practitioner lens as well as the workforce development opportunity for practitioners to undertake research as part of their daily practice, was also a key driver for the model.

Understanding research in a local authority

Whilst the co-production evaluation programme was established within the PCT the work became operational post transfer into local authority in 2013. Within the NHS there are very clear protocols and guidance for research and development but within local government this is less clear cut. It was agreed with the R&D lead within local government that university ethics would be accepted as the approved process for the work and the standard template for R&D to be logged in local government would also be completed and recorded.

Sharing co-production evaluation learning and publication

One of the key aspirations of the co-production evaluation programme has always been to achieve publication within peer-reviewed journals. The opportunity for public health practitioners to develop the skills and competence to undertake quality assured evaluations and subsequently participate in the development of a peer reviewed journal article is not something often available at practitioner level.

During the course of the co-production evaluation journey there have been many opportunities to submit poster presentations to conferences such as Public Health England conference. These conferences are expensive to attend and often the cost renders them prohibitive for public health practitioners. Participating in co-produced evaluations with the embedded researcher has opened doors for practitioners to attend these conferences and share their learning with broader audiences.

What are the key lessons learnt?

Finding the right academic

This process is not for all researchers. It is a very pragmatic way to test the evidence base and determine how well it is being implemented within the field. With a small budget allocation the embedded researcher is often relatively junior in their academic career and so it is essential there is a professor with robust oversight and scrutiny of the work. The passion to bring academic skills into the front line work of public health and the opportunity to publish small-scale evaluations to add to the richness and diversity of the evidence base requires a true belief in translational research.

Screening for eligible projects (ensure there is baseline data)

The programmes / interventions put forward for evaluation must meet a set criteria to warrant the evaluation viable. All public health practitioners receive the following guidance when submitting a request to participate in a co-production evaluation:

> It is important to note that these are co-production pieces of work with researchers from Teesside University. By completing these forms you are agreeing to be involved in all areas of the research and the work to be divided between yourself and the researcher. This is worked out at the beginning of the individual projects and will need to be agreed by line managers. Please complete the relevant form below relating to the methodological area. The forms will be shortlisted by DCC and then Professor Newbury-Birch will identify which proposals are the most academically sound. At this stage we will have a meeting with yourself and if an implementation or evaluation study we will meet with the providers also to ensure the extent of the data that can be collected in order to carry out the study and work out the correct methodological framework that is needed in order to do the study.

Clarity of roles and responsibilities

To ensure all public health senior management team had a full appreciation of the commitment to undertake a co-produced evaluation the following roles and responsibilities agreement was constructed (Table 1.1).

Embedding R&D objectives into practitioner work plans

To fully reflect the work to be undertaken the co-production evaluation must be fully recognised within the job plan of the practitioner. This demonstrates corporate commitment to the time needed to complete the work and learn from the process.

Timeline for intervention

Timelines inevitably waver slightly due to ethics or the coordination of focus groups or a myriad of other legitimate reasons. However, wherever possible the evaluations are completed within a 12-month period.

Table 1.1 Role clarity

Aspect of evaluation	University responsibilities	Durham County Council Responsibilities
Induction	**Spend one half day each shadowing the other in their day job (time permitting) to get to know each other better and to understand their roles.**	
Steering groups	Note taking for the meetings	Identification of steering group members
		Chairing of steering group
	The arranging of dates and times for steering group meetings and the setting of the agenda will be a joint responsibility	
	Roles and responsibilities of the wider steering group will be discussed and decided upon depending on the needs of the evaluation. Additionally a steering group is held once a quarter to discuss co-production work and share learning amongst the public health leads and university staff.	
Evaluation protocol	Conduct basic literature review outlining evidence for teen parent programmes and their impact on well-being and future employment.	Provide expertise on national and local policy relating to their portfolio
	Design initial protocol including combined literature review, and proposed methods for data collection and analysis	Provide feedback on the initial protocol for the final draft.
	Evaluation protocol to be shared with the steering group once finalised for comments	
Governance	Take lead on university ethics application – to be completed prior to any data being shared with the university	Take lead on Durham research application pack and any Caldecott agreements needed to share data with Teesside University. Liaise with necessary people at Council.
Data collection and analysis	TO BE COMPLETED FOR EACH PROJECT	
Final report	Background section of report to be shared between. University will take lead on writing up the literature search. DCC to take the lead on writing up of current national and local policy relevant to their portfolio.	
	Take the lead on writing up the methodology section of the report.	Take lead on participant recruitment section of the methodology
	Provide feedback on sections of the Methodology written by DCC.	Provide feedback on the Methods section written by University

Do not over commit

In the first wave of evaluations there were five evaluations undertaken. This became unmanageable for the researcher and also if the practitioner was participating in more than one evaluation project there became a pressure on capacity to undertake other work objectives. It was agreed after the first wave of evaluations that an researcher would not run more than three evaluations and any single practitioner would only commit to one.

Understanding political landscape and changing/emerging priorities

At a time of significant national austerity and political uncertainty of the public health grant many public health interventions are at risk of being de-commissioned due to the necessity to prioritise programme areas. A couple of co-produced evaluations undertaken helped to make commissioning decisions regarding the future delivery of the programmes and the opportunity cost of money being invested elsewhere. During the process it may have felt complex and uncertain for the embedded researcher who was not familiar with working in this political environment but again this is back to research being completed in the context of local. In the real world of local authority work programmes are vulnerable, complex, uncertain and ambiguous (VUCA).

Contributing to the evidence base – local priorities and local relevance

The work undertaken over the last few years has resulted in poster and oral presentations at regional, national and international conferences and to date and seven co-produced publications (McGeechan et al. 2016a; McGeechan et al. 2016b; McGeechan et al. 2016c; McGeechan et al. 2018a; McGeechan et al. 2018b; McGeechan et al. 2018c; McGeechan in press). This has enabled the co-production evaluation programme to raise its profile and demonstrate the added value of small scale evaluations being conducted in the context of local authority public health teams which is of relevance to local level priorities.

References

Glasgow, R. E., E. Lichtenstein and A. C. Marcus (2003). "Why don't we see more translation of health promotion research to practice?" *Am J Public Health* 93(8): 1261–1267.

Hemming, K., T. P. Haines, P. J. Chilton, A. J. Girling and R. J. Lilford (2015). "The stepped wedge cluster randomised trial: rationale, design, analysis, and reporting." *BMJ: British Medical Journal* 350: h391.

May, C. and T. Finch (2009). "Implementation, embedding, and integration: an outline of Normalization Process Theory." *Sociology* 43(3): 535–554.

McGeechan, G. J., C. Richardson, K. Weir, L. Wilson, G. O'Neill and D. Newbury-Birch, (2018a). "Evaluation of a police led suicide early alert surveillance strategy in the United Kingdom." *Injury Prevention* 24: 267–271.

McGeechan, G., D. Phillips, L. Wilson, V. J. Whittaker, G. O'Neill, and D. Newbury-Birch (2018b). "Service evaluation of an exercise on referral scheme for adults with existing health conditions in the United Kingdom." *International J Behav Med* 25: 304–311.

McGeechan, G., C. Richardson, L. Wilson, G. O'Neill, and D. Newbury-Birch (2016a). "Exploring men's perceptions of a community based men's shed programme in England." *Journal of Public Health* 39(4): e251–e256.

McGeechan, G., K. Wilkinson, N. Martin, L. Wilson, G. O'Neill and D. Newbury-Birch (2016b). "A mixed method outcome evaluation of a specialist Alcohol Hospital Liaison Team." *Perspectives in Public Health* 136(6): 361–367.

McGeechan, G., D. Woodhall, L. Anderson, L. Wilson, G. O'Neill and D. Newbury-Birch (2016c). "A coproduction community based approach to reducing smoking prevalence in a local community setting." *Journal of Environmental and Public Health*: 538–653.

McGeechan G. J., M. Baldwin, K. Allan, G. O'Neill, and D. Newbury-Birch (2018c). "Exploring young women's perspectives of a targeted support programme for teenage parents." *BMJ Sexual & Reproductive Health* 44(4): 272–277.

McGeechan, G. J., C. Richardson, L. Wilson, K. Allan, and D. Newbury-Birch. "A qualitative exploration of a school based mindfulness course for young people." *Child and Adolescent Mental Health.*

Michie, S., D. Fixsen, J. M. Grimshaw and M. P. Eccles (2009). "Specifying and reporting complex behaviour change interventions: the need for a scientific method." *Implementation Science* 4(1): 40.

Morris, Z., S. Wooding and J. Grant (2011). "The answer is 17 years, what is the question: understanding time lags in translational research." *Journal of the Royal Society of Medicine* 104(12): 510–520.

Newbury-Birch, D., G. McGeechan and A. Holloway (2016). "Climbing down the steps from the ivory tower: how UK academics and criminal justice practitioners need to work together on alcohol studies." *International Journal of Prisoner Health* 12(3): 129–134.

Petticrew, M., S. Cummins, C. Ferrell, A. Findlay, C. Higgins, C. Hoy, A. Kearns and L. Sparks (2005). "Natural experiments: an underused tool for public health?" *Public Health* 119(9): 751–757.

2 Co-production

The academic perspective

Grant J. McGeechan, Louisa J. Ells and Emma L. Giles

As a delivery model for health and social care, co-production has been described as sharing information and decision making between service users and providers (Realpe and Wallace 2010), which when effectively applied can improve services, and enable service users to become more effective agents of change (Penny et al. 2012). However, this model is increasingly used to bring together academics, policy makers and communities to produce research that is not only academically excellent but importantly has real public benefit. In this chapter we will examine the co-production endeavour from the academic researcher's point of view. We will consider the barriers and facilitators to effective co-production in academia, drawing on many years of practice experience. This chapter will feature interviews with researchers in order to capture their opinions around the unique opportunities afforded by co-production work.

Background

The primary goal of any public health research is to improve the health and wellbeing of our target communities. However, too often there appears to be a disjunction between public health research and public health policy and practice; with lengthy delays between the evidence generation and translation (Morris et al. 2011), and difficulties in implementing evidence generated from highly controlled experiments within complex real world settings (Kemm 2006). Within research the often perceived gold standard in study design is the randomised controlled trial (RCT) (Kaptchuk 2001). Whilst many readers may be familiar with the premise of an RCT, for those of you who are not, then, briefly, these involve a tightly controlled experimental study designed to compare two or more groups of things (people, objects, chemicals, elements) when exposed to a particular variable to see if there is any difference in how they respond to that variable once exposed to it. However, in reality once an intervention is delivered in a real-world setting there are often a number of variables at play that cannot be controlled, and often mean that results cannot be replicated once rolled out to the general public (Pettman et al. 2012).

Additionally, whilst many will view academics and practitioners as coming from different worlds, in actuality the boundaries are blurred (Wehrens 2014). It has been proposed that a co-production approach involving academics and practitioners working together will result in services that better translate into real world practice and are more meaningful to those who will engage with them (Graham and Tetroe 2007).

There are many different names for co-production research (Graham et al. 2006) such as knowledge translation (Straus et al. 2009; Davis et al. 2003; Grimshaw et al. 2012), participatory action research (Whyte 1991; McIntyre 2007), and collaborative research (Bloedon and Stokes 1994), which can vary greatly in methodology depending on the area of interest. However, most tend to adhere to similar principles, where the exchange, synthesis, and dissemination of knowledge between researchers, policy makers, practitioners and end users is key (Tetroe 2007). There are a number of different theoretical approaches to co-production research, for example Straus and colleagues (Straus et al. 2009) developed the knowledge to action framework, which can be utilised at all levels of translational research from the local to global level. Within this model is a clearly defined process for knowledge creation that may be useful for asset-based health research consisting of three key phases: knowledge inquiry, synthesis of knowledge, and creation of knowledge tools. Knowledge inquiry includes the completion of primary research, whilst synthesis of knowledge includes bringing together research findings relevant to the topic. The final stage involves further synthesis of the best quality knowledge into decision-making tools, policy and practice guidelines, or delivery of services.

In the book *Beyond two communities: the co-production of research, policy and practice in collaborative public health settings* (Morris et al. 2011) Wehrens identifies four distinct approaches to co-production between practitioners responsible for delivering services and university academics. Each model differs in the level of integration between both sets of professionals, and how meaning is constructed within the partnership. The four approaches are: Boundary Organisations, Hybrid Management, Front and Back Stage regions, and Communities of Practice.

Boundary Organisations was first posited by Guston (Guston 1999). This theoretical approach to co-production work draws on a socio-political perspective of boundary work and political approaches to agent theory. A unique component of boundary organisations within the wider literature on co-production is that each partner continues to negotiate the different social worlds in which they operate, however they remain accountable to their host organisation only. As such, whilst there will be a degree of compromise and commonality on the goals of the co-production work being undertaken, each partner will retain the pressures, and competing priorities of their own organisation, whilst trying to satisfy the needs of the project.

Hybrid Management emerged as an adaption of the boundary organisation approach, first proposed by Miller (Miller 2001), which moved away from the socio-political foundations of boundary organisations, instead focussing on the practices within an academic and policy making partnership. Whilst within a boundary organisation approach each party retains a large degree of autonomy from one another, with a hybrid management approach partners are sufficiently intertwined so as to remove the possibility for autonomy. Within this approach, Miller outlines four key processes that facilitate hybrid management. First, there needs to be a sufficient level of integration between academic and practice elements of the project; this is to ensure that they are speaking the same language (hybridisation). However, it is also essential to deconstruct these elements so that any underlying assumptions can be addressed (deconstruction). However, whilst autonomy should be impossible due to integration between academic and practice partners, there should still be clearly defined boundaries (boundary work) so that each partner knows which aspects of the project they are responsible for (cross-domain orchestration).

Front stage and backstage regions, first proposed by Goffman (Goffman 1990) looks at the distinction between how co-production work is presented to front stage and backstage audiences. The front stage is defined as those not directly involved in the project, such as members of the public or interested stakeholders, whilst those in the backstage are those partners directly involved in the project. According to this theory there is a distinct difference between the messages portrayed to each audience, the front stage audience receive a performance that suggests that the project embodies certain standards. The backstage, on the other hand, is reserved for insiders involved in the project, where the 'performance' is deliberately contradicted.

Communities of practice: The final approach proposed by Wenger, McDermott, and Snyder (Wenger et al. 2002) deviates slightly from the other approaches. Within this approach, partners come together because they share a passion about a particular topic, and whilst they come from different backgrounds they are able to draw on their collective strengths to deepen their individual knowledge, and achieve the project aims.

The above approaches provide a useful framework for conducting co-production work, although in practice it can be difficult to adhere to any one approach. However, evidence suggests that when co-production is employed, it can be an effective approach (Sherman et al. 2015). For example, a number of academics and practitioners who have contributed to various chapters of this book have been involved in long-running co-production projects centred on the evaluation of locally commissioned public health services, and providing national policy and practice support. Whilst the theoretical approach most closely aligned to these projects could be described as communities of practice, one could also argue that it incorporates elements of boundary organisations and hybrid management as well. Whilst each partner retains a degree of autonomy, and reports to their host organisation, there is also a degree of integration achieved through a researcher in residence model, which allows each partner to learn from each other, and use their collective knowledge to achieve the aims of the evaluation. Whilst the effectiveness of these project will be for others to judge, we feel that there have been a number of benefits, as well as some hurdles, from these long running project, some of which will be summarised below.

Limitations and strengths

As with most forms of research there are both limitations and strengths to co-production. From an academic perspective it is very common to disseminate research via journal publication. However, the goal of practitioners is often more about evidence-based practice, with a target audience who may not routinely use, or indeed have access to, peer reviewed journals. Therefore, co-production research may be more about sharing the skills, knowledge, and experience of both the researcher and practitioner. Whilst the goal may not necessarily be to produce journal publications, this is not to say that this is impossible. In fact, many co-produced projects result in publication. However, it is important to consider who needs to know, what they need to know, and what are the most appropriate mechanisms to reach your target audience. This may result in several different publications, with a different focus for different audiences. For example, the authors' co-production projects with local authority practitioners have resulted in numerous publications (McGeehan et al. 2016, 2017, 2018). Further examples include the co-production of: the standard evaluation framework for weight management intervention (website and peer review publication) (Ells et al. 2013, 2017); evidence to support the national sugar reduction strategy (report and peer review publication) (Ells et al. 2015; Roberts et al. 2017) and the national weight management commissioning toolkit (Coulton et al. 2017) and supporting video (Teesside University Digital Studio 2017). However, once published, a hurdle may be that readers may not perceive such publications as 'robust' research (Martin 2010). It could be that they are perceived to fall short of the 'gold standard' of a RCT (Kaptchuk 2001), as they tend to be more pragmatic, real-life evaluations of existing services, with limited scope for researchers to shape the study design. This must not, however, detract from the importance of publishing. So long as the strengths and limitations of the study design are appropriately articulated, evidence from service evaluations can provide an important contribution to the evidence base. This evidence can document valuable insights into what works and what does not in real world setting, often providing critical learning about evidence implementation and outcomes from harder to reach communities who would be unlikely to participate in traditional trials.

Co-production projects can be tricky; as with any industry, stakeholders working together face a number of challenges. For academics, competing priorities can include funding priorities, teaching and learning responsibilities, continuing professional development, and leadership and administrative duties. For practitioners, their priorities could include delivering a cost-effective service within the confines of an ever-changing public health climate and, sometimes, within restricted budgetary and time constraints. This can mean that from both sides, time is limited to a truly co-produced – balanced – approach, with one side having to take the lead at any one time to drive-forward the project, but with an underlying mutual respect and equality in relationship that is fundamental to successful co-production.

A further challenge to co-production with public health practitioners, can be the alignment between evaluation or research timeframes and commissioning cycles or policy/practice deadlines. Additionally, practitioners may be disinclined to work with academics for fear of detrimental findings that may suggest service decommissioning, or vice versa. The evidence may suggest that the service is effective, but a decision has already been made to decommission the service due to budgetary constraints. This can lead to tensions between stakeholders, as the service can be decommissioned before the evaluation can be completed. On the other hand, the results of the evaluation may not conform to the practitioner's pre-existing views of the effectiveness/ value of that service. However, in practice these challenges are overcome through a shared focus on improving population health, and effective communication with all relevant stakeholders to ensure all expectations are managed from the projects inception. The use of evaluability assessments (such as that described by Davies (2013)) and standard evaluation frameworks (such as the Public Health England weight management framework (Ells et al. 2017)), can be very helpful in bringing together all stakeholders, and ensuring all expectations for the evaluation are managed from the outset.

Whilst there are limitations to co-production work, the strengths far outweigh the limitations when successful co-production is undertaken. Take, for example, a local authority with a long running weight management service. The local authority will need to know: is the service cost and clinically effective, is it reaching its target population, and is the service fit for purpose, yet there is often no capacity and or expertise in house to undertake the required evaluation. Through a commissioned co-produced academic evaluation, the local authority will gain a range of different skills and expertise delivered by the academic team, and a rigorous independent evaluation, which will help inform future service improvements and commissioning decisions. The academic will gain valuable insight into real-world service delivery, with opportunities to analyse novel datasets and access populations who may otherwise be hard to reach. These opportunities provide invaluable shared learning, which can lead to ongoing co-production through collaborative research bids to address real world questions that have arisen from the evaluation.

Practitioners also provide access to a local authority 'brand', which could mean that participants are more trusting and willing to engage with evaluations. For example, as part of one of our evaluations of an alcohol service it transpired that participants involved in the service had not provided consent for their data to be shared. They had to then be retrospectively contacted by the service providers to give consent for their data to be used. After being contacted, the clear majority agreed for their data to be used. This could be because the public respond well to practitioners, arguably less well to academics (Michael 2000). This may not have been as successful should they have been cold-called by academics only.

Whilst we have detailed a number of strengths for academics working on co-production projects, we also hope that there are positives for our partners working in practice, indeed many of them have told us that they have found the process enlightening. In particular, working with academic partners provides them with the opportunity to share their expertise, knowledge, and hopefully evidence of good practice with a wider audience. One of the central components to co-production in our view is the sharing of knowledge and expertise; with this in mind we offer practitioners the opportunity to assist in the drafting of scientific publications, and conference abstracts. Over the years we have built up a portfolio of scientific publications that include public health practitioners as co-authors (McGeechan et al. 2016, 2017, 2018; Ells et al. 2018; Roberts et al. 2017). However, as academics we are also provided with the opportunity to write lay and practice-based reports, supported by our policy practice partners and or service users. This cross learning contributes to the professional development of both academic and policy practice partners and ensures that learning from co-produced work reaches the widest possible audiences, thus maximised the potential public health impact.

Central to many of our co-production projects has been the implementation of the embedded researcher or researcher/practitioner in residence approach, whereby honorary contracts are held with partner organisations. This provides each party an opportunity to embed themselves within collaborating organisations. Practitioners have found space within the university useful in terms of building networks, and providing protected time for space writing and access to supporting scientific publications. For the academics it has provided a critical opportunity to be immersed within policy/practice culture: building networks and understanding the procedures, processes and pressures of partner organisations. We feel that this approach gives both academics and practitioners critical insight and appreciation each other's organisational pressures, as well as some protected time and space to dedicate to the co-production project.

Pressure points

Whilst co-production projects result in many positive outcomes, there can be pressure points. One of these pressure points concerns is ethical approvals. Whilst not required for literature reviews, any primary research, service evaluations or secondary data analysis coproduced with a university introduces an additional process to acquire university ethics and research governance approval. This process is required in addition to governance approvals from partner organisations, which can add to the project timetable. However, these processes are necessary to ensure that all work is undertaken legally and ethically, but it is important to be upfront with co-production partners about the potential time implications of these processes at the start of the project before any timelines are agreed.

An additional pressure point concerns the practicalities of running a project, such as organising honorary contracts and administrative support. Often projects require logistics input, for example to organise steering committee meetings, sort and deliver information packs to participants, or transcribe audio recordings. It is therefore important to establish at the start of a project, which organisation will take responsibility for which administrative tasks. It is therefore prudent to work together from the start to develop a detailed project plan with clear lines of responsibility, and initial the necessary processes for honorary contracts at the earliest opportunity.

One further pressure point is the conflict between timescales, robustness, and speed. Often policy and practice projects have tight deadlines to meet, which are linked to commissioning timescales and national policy demands. These can be short term, requiring flexibility and speed to accommodate change. This need-for-speed can be at odds with traditional academic methods, which whilst thorough can often be long and drawn-out (Martin 2010). Therefore, careful negotiation may be required up-front to be open and honest around how long different phases of the research may take, and when milestones can feasibly be achieved, and deliverables provided. It may be necessary to use different methodologies in order to meet policy or practice needs, and if these differ from the academic gold standard, the limitations of the more pragmatic approach, and the impact this may have on the interpretation of the findings must be clearly articulated. Whilst ideally a co-production project would involve an equal partnership, when time pressures arise, the academic partner is often required to take on the bulk of the work to ensure that projects remain on track (Martin 2010).

Case study

To illustrate the impact of co-production, we highlight a case study from Professor Ells' applied obesity research programme at Teesside University. Having previously co-founded the National Obesity Observatory, Professor Ells returned to academia to establish a translational research programme to address the real-world public health priorities that she had seen emerging from policy and practice. Driven by a shared passion and commitment to make a real and tangible difference to population health, she has worked in co-production with a number of key strategic local, national and international stakeholders. This includes:

* working in co-production with the European Association for the Study of Obesity to provide evidence based training on the treatment of child and adolescent obesity.
* undertaking a longstanding part-time secondment with Public Health England (PHE), which continues to provide invaluable first-hand

experience of the needs, expectations, and constraints of local and national policy and practice. Resulting coproduced products include an update of the standard evaluation framework for weight management interventions (Ells et al. 2017), a report mapping national weight management services (Coulton et al. 2015), a report examining weight status tracking during primary school (Copley et al. 2017), and supporting the production of the PHE weight management commissioner and provider toolkits (Teesside University Digital Studio 2017). Professor Ells' team also led evidence reviews that helped inform the 2015 PHE national sugar reduction strategy (Tedstone et al. 2015); as well as the implementation and evaluation of a Teesside University sugar reduction tax and marketing campaign, which was show cased as a national case study (Tedstone et al. 2015).

* working in co-production with local authorities to undertake weight management service evaluations that have directly informed service improvements and commissioning decisions.

Key to these successful co-production projects have been:

* the establishment of good mutually respectful relationships with policy and practice partners.
* appreciating the needs, constraints and expectations of policy and practice partners, and working flexibly and pragmatically to accommodate these, whilst maintaining the highest possible quality and academic integrity of all outputs.
* ensuring open lines of communication, supported by detailed project plans with clear lines of responsibility, milestones and realistic timeframes from the start of every project. It is vitally important that all projects are delivered on time and to the required specifications.
* publishing findings using a range of different methods including reports, peer review publications, lay summaries, infographics and film, to maximise the reach and impact of products.
* ensuring all relevant stakeholders are engaged and valued throughout the co-production process.

Changes to practice

One of the fundamental reasons for undertaking co-production research is the ability to influence policy and practice. Not only can research provide academic benefits, such as an original contribution to the wider literature, but it can offer wider benefits to policy. This is particularly highlighted in the case study above, which clearly shows how co-produced work can have a positive impact on policy. This, in turn, can translate into benefits for practice, with obvious examples being medical research, which can become embedded in

National Institute for Health and Care Excellence (NICE) guidance, and therefore change on-the-ground disease treatment, for example. Co-produced research can also be used to influence service commissioning within local authorities, which, in turn, can bring real change in communities, with for example, access to facilities and support groups, that otherwise may not exist for individuals and their families.

One of the key questions that co-production researchers may ask themselves is 'how can we make a difference'? Some research can be very focused on theory, often perhaps described as 'ivory tower' research, and which can be far removed from the world of practice and even individual life. That is not to say that such research isn't required, but the key strength of co-production research, and aspirations of co-production researchers, is that their research has real-world application, and is picked up and used by those who would most benefit from it (Newbury-Birch et al. 2016). Making a positive change for the lives of individuals, groups, and communities is fundamental, particularly from a public health co-production perspective.

Top five tips

- Co-production relates to the exchange, synthesis, and dissemination of knowledge between researchers, policymakers, and end users.
- It benefits both academics and practitioners, and can result in valuable shared learning.
- Pressure points can cause conflict, but can be overcome through well-discussed and thought-through projects.
- Making real-world change is often the result of good co-produced research.
- There are benefits to multiple stakeholders, including academics, practitioners, policy makers, and the general public, from co-produced research.

References

Bloedon, R.V. and Stokes, D.R. Making university/industry collaborative research succeed. *Research-Technology Management*. 1994;37(2):44–48.

Bloedon, R.V. and Stokes, D.R., Copley, V., Ells, L., Brya, C., Strugnell, C., Mead, E., Taylor, R., Manners, R., Johal, G., and Perkins, C.Making university/industry collaborative research succeed. *Research-Technology Management*. 1994;37:44–48.

Copley, V., Ells, L., Bray, C., Strugnell, C., Mead, E., Taylor, R., Manners, R., Johal, G., and Perkins, C. *Changes in the weight status of children between the first and final years of primary school*. London: Public Health England; 2017 p. 57.

Coulton, V., Dodhia, S., Ells, L., and Blackshaw, J. *National mapping of weight management services*. London: Public Health England; 2015 p. 37.

Coulton, V., Ells, L., Blackshaw, J., Boylan, E., and Tedstone, A. *A guide to delivering and commissioning tier 2 weight management services for children and their families*

[Internet]. Public Health England; 2017 [cited 2018 Sep 21] p. 47. Available from: https://assets.publishing.service.gov.uk/government/uploads/system/uploads/attachm ent_data/file/649196/tier2_child_weight_management_services_guide.pdf

Coulton, V., Dodhia, S., Ells, L., and Blackshaw, J. *National mapping of weight management services.* Public Health England; 2015 p. 37.

Davies, R. *Planning evaluability assessments: A synthesis of the literature with recommendations.* [Internet]. Department for International Development; 2013 [cited 2018 Sep 21]. Available from: https://www.gov.uk/dfid-research-outputs/planning-evalua bility-assessments-a-synthesis-of-the-literature-with-recommendations-dfid-working-paper-40

Davis, D., Davis, M.E., Jadad, A., Rath, D., Ryan, D., Sibbald, G., Straus, S., Rappolt, S., Wowk, M., and Zwarenstein, M. The case for knowledge translation: shortening the journey from evidence to effect. *BMJ.* 2003;327:33–35.

Ells, L.J., Cavill, N., Roberts, K., and Rutter, H. Development of a Standard Evaluation Framework for Weight Management Interventions. *Public Health.* 2013;127:345–347.

Ells, L., Roberts, K., McGowan, V., and Machaira, T. *Sugar reduction: The evidence for action Annexe 2: A mixed method review of behaviour changes resulting from experimental studies that examine the effect of fiscal measures targeted at high sugar food and non-alcoholic drink* [Internet]. Public Health England; 2015 [cited 2018 Sep 21] p. 87. Available from: https://assets.publishing.service.gov.uk/government/uploa ds/system/uploads/attachment_data/file/470173/Annexe_2._Fiscal_evidence_review. pdf

Ells, L., Roberts, K., and Cavil, N. *Standard evaluation framework for weight management interventions* [Internet]. Public Health England; 2017 [cited 2018 Sep 21] p. 57. Available from: https://assets.publishing.service.gov.uk/government/uploads/ system/uploads/attachment_data/file/685545/SEF_weight_management_interven tions.pdf

Ells, L., Watson, P., Carlebach, S., O'Malley, C., Jones, D., Machaira, T., Whittaker, V., Clements, H., Walker, P., Needham, K., Summerbell, C., Coulton, V., and Araujo-Soares, V. A mixed method evaluation of adult tier 2 lifestyle weight management service provision across a county in Northern England. *Clinical Obesity.* 2018, Apr 24;8(3):191–202.

Goffman, E. *The presentation of self in everyday life. 8th ed.* London: Penguin; 1990.

Graham, I.D., Logan, J., Harrison, M.B., Straus, S.E., Tetroe, J., Caswell, W., and Robinson, N.Lost in knowledge translation: time for a map? *Journal of Continuing Education in the Health Professions.* 2006;26:13–24.

Graham, I.D. and Tetroe, J. How to translate health research knowledge into effective healthcare action. *Health CQ.* 2007;10(3):20–22.

Grimshaw, J.M., Eccles, M.P., Lavis, J.N., Hill, S.J., and Squires, J.E. Knowledge translation of research findings. *Implementation Science.* 2012;7:50.

Guston, D.H. Stabilizing the boundary between US politics and science: The role of the Office of Technology Transfer as a boundary organization *Social Studies of Science.* 1999;29:87–111.

Kaptchuk, T.J. The double-blind, randomized, placebo-controlled trial: Gold standard or golden calf? *Journal of Clinical Epidemiology.* 2001Jun 1;54(6):541–549.

Kemm, J. The limitations of 'evidence-based' public health. *Journal of Evaluation in Clinical Practice.* 2006, May 22;12(3):319–324.

Martin, S. Co-production of social research: Strategies for engaged scholarship. *Public Money & Management.* 2010;(4):211–218.

McGeechan, G.J., Wilkinson, K.G., Martin, N., Wilson, L., and Newbury-Birch, D. A mixed method outcome evaluation of a specialist Alcohol Hospital Liaison Team. *Perspectives in Public Health.* 2016;136:361–367.

McGeechan, G.J., Richardson, C., Wilson, L., O'Neill, G., and Newbury-Birch, D. Exploring men's perceptions of a community-based men's shed programme in England *Journal of Public Health.* 2017, Dec 1;39(4):e251–256.

McGeechan, G., Richardson, C., Wilson, L., Allan, K., and Newbury-Birch, D. A qualitative exploration of a school based mindfulness course for young people *Child and Adolescent Mental Health.* 2018;24(2):154–160.

McIntyre, A. *Participatory action research. Vol. 52.* Thousand Oaks, CA: Sage Publications; 2007.

Michael, J. *Anxious intellects: Academic professionals, public intellectuals, and enlightenment values.* Durham, NC: Duke University Press; 2000.

Miller, C. Hybrid management: boundary organizations, science policy, and environmental governance in the climate regime. *Science, Technology, & Human Values.* 2001;26:478–500.

Morris, Z.S., Wooding, S., and Grant, J. The answer is 17 years, what is the question: Understanding time lags in translational research. *J R Soc Med.* 2011Dec;104 (12):510–520.

Newbury-Birch, D., McGeechan, G.J., and Holloway, A. Climbing down the steps from the ivory tower: How UK academics and criminal justice practitioners need to work together on alcohol studies. *International Journal of Prisoner Health.* 2016, Sep 12;12(3):129–134.

Penny, J., Slay, J., and Stephens, L. *People powered health co-production catalogue.* London: NEF/NESTA; 2012.

Pettman, T.L., Armstrong, R., Doyle, J., Burford, B., Anderson, L.M., Hilgrove, T., Honey, N., and Waters, H.E. Strengthening evaluation to capture the breadth of public health practice: Ideal vs. real. *Journal of Public Health.* 2012; 37:151–155.

Realpe, A. and Wallace, L. *What is co-production?* [Internet]. The Health Foundation; 2010 [cited 2018 Sep 21]. Available from: http://personcentredcare.health.org.uk/sites/default/files/resources/what_is_co-production.pdf

Roberts, K.E., Ells, L.J., McGowan, V.J., Machaira, T., Targett, V.C., Allen, R.E., and Tedstone, A.E.A rapid review examining purchasing changes resulting from fiscal measures targeted at high sugar foods and sugar-sweetened drinks. Nutrition & Diabetes [Internet]. 2017, Dec [cited 2018 Sep 21];7(12). Available from: http://www.nature.com/articles/s41387-017-0001-1

Sherman, L.W., Strang, H., Barnes, G., Woods, D.J., Bennett, S., Inkpen, N., Newbury-Birch, D., Rossner, M., Angel, C., Mearns., and Slothower, M. Twelve experiments in restorative justice: The Jerry Lee program of randomized trials of restorative justice conferences. *J Exp Criminol.* 2015, Dec 1;11(4):501–540.

Straus, S.E., Tetroe, J., and Graham, I. Defining knowledge translation. *Canadian Medical Association Journal.* 2009;181:165–168.

Tedstone, A., Targett, V., and Allen, R. *Sugar reduction: The evidence for action.* London: Public Health England; 2015 p. 48.

Teesside University Digital Studio. *Introduction to the weight management guide* [Internet] Teesside University Digital Studio; 2017 [cited 2018 Sep 21]. (Weight management: guidance for commissioners and providers). Available from: https://

www.gov.uk/government/collections/weight-management-guidance-for-commissio
ners-and-providers

Tetroe, J. Knowledge translation at the Canadian Institutes of Health Research: A
primer. *Focus Tech Brief.* 2007;1–8.

Wehrens, R. Beyond two communities – from research utilization and knowledge
translation to co-production? *Public Health.* 2014;128:545–551.

Wenger, E., McDermott, R.A., and Snyder, W. *Cultivating communities of practice: A
guide to managing knowledge.* Boston: Harvard Business Press; 2002.

Whyte, W.F. *Participatory action research.* Newbury-Park: Sage Publications; 1991.

3 Co-production

The public health practitioner's perspective

Keith Allan, Michelle Baldwin, Kirsty Wilkinson and Dianne Woodall

Co-production is, when working well, a mutualistic relationship between two or more parties in which expertise is shared to gain greater insight to address an issue. In terms of co-production between public health practitioner and researcher an academic's focus may be on developing publications and adding to the sum of scientific knowledge the practitioner in turn may have their attention fixed upon development and evaluation of a fitter service. While these do not represent exactly the same aims they are not mutually exclusive and there can be benefits for both sides. There is, however, the potential for tension, discomfort and irritation as differing pressures, timescales and philosophies meet.

An important first step in creating a useful co-production relationship is to be clear about the purpose of the project. It is important to be clear from the outset, from a practitioner point of view, what is needed for an individual service (e.g. what needs to be monitored or assessed to demonstrate potential outcomes that may be contracted for with the service provider) and what the intended purpose of working with an academic is. The importance of that word, "with" cannot be overstated. There needs to be a clear understanding that the incoming academic is there to add value and usually to provide some form of rigorous assessment during the project but they have not simply been contracted to provide an audit or to simply be an additional set of hands. Reciprocally it should be made clear that the practitioners are not just sources of data or in the role of research assistant but that the project is truly collaborative. The main purpose of co-production, as seen from the practitioner's point of view can range from designing and developing more robust evaluations to developing the skills of the practitioner team within the research. The provision of academic rigour and the effect that the inclusion of a co-production project into a work stream has can serve to raise the planning and profile of a service so that evaluation is not relegated to being an afterthought.

Co-production can have benefits for the individual practitioner, allowing them to practically apply tools and techniques learnt elsewhere, for example as part of their own studies. Furthermore, it can be seen as an opportunity to generate high-quality evidence for future work due to the extra level of sense checking and adherence to agreed standard operating procedures. The access to both academic expertise and software were both seen as potential benefits to practitioners. Additionally, working with an academic can add credibility when engaging with a range of stakeholder groups such as health promotion professionals, members of the community and senior management or community leaders.

However, there are costs to this approach; the need to proceed in an academically robust fashion can introduce an additional time cost. To facilitate the integration of operational teams and researchers additional meetings and governance structures are often created. This can be variable between institutions, for example local authorities or NHS. In addition there is further need to arrange for time to be given over to support access between the academic and operational team. Similarly, there is the opportunity cost reflected in the practitioner's time within the co-production model. In the more familiar commissioning model one would expect to hand off a significant portion of the work to be done to the incoming partner. This use of resource, in terms of funds paid to the commissioned party, allows the practitioner to work on other projects and perhaps hold a more supervisory role in the commissioned project. This is not the case with co-production. Instead there may be more significant calls on the practitioner's time as they work collaboratively with the academic.

In discussions with practitioners gaining the experience of academics was highly valued but so was the opportunity to demonstrate their own expertise. Furthermore, the relationship was valued for its peer support, working to each other's strengths and supporting one another when the best course of action may have been unclear. Practitioners also highlighted the benefit in findings being less questionable if they had been developed with an academic, especially when their specialist skills in research methods were used.

Practitioners also point out their value to the academics; this essentially allowed easier and more efficient access to their host organisation. This may include governance arrangements, writing management reports and undertaking presentations to convey the findings in a context relevant for the organisation. Indeed, it is possible for a practitioner to gain useful experience and exposure within their own organisation in the process. This also links to the benefit of being able to translate important academic findings directly into actions understood and appreciated by management teams, ultimately to the public's benefit.

There were also additional benefits to some practitioners as the experience of working with academics was also useful to them in terms of continual professional development and pursuing their own training, such as developing new skills in a given research method, and higher education. Furthermore expectations for the reach of assessments may be strengthened during the co-production process. For example, if a more traditional approach is taken to service evaluation there would be little expectation of presenting anything beyond a performance report based upon agreed key performance indicators.

However, when the priorities of an academic are also included it can mean that practitioners also gain by having the opportunity to contribute to the body of scientific literature in a way that they may not otherwise.

There can be a number of complications to the relationship, however. Both universities and delivery organisations have their own hierarchies, governance bodies and normal procedures. It is natural to assume that the procedures of the organisation one belongs to would take precedence. To avoid conflicts later in the process it is important that these issues are scoped out early in the process and a protocol agreed by all stakeholders. There are often ethical considerations that may not have been apparent within a single organisation but are generated when university and host organisation come together. This may include what data can and cannot be used for and where it may be viewed. It is likely that data will be available for service monitoring, performance and development but may not, due to issues of consent, be initially available for pure research. This raised awareness of consent and the need to build it into data capture is another strong benefit of co-production between academic and practitioner.

There can be some deleterious aspects of this form of co-production. It requires a greater time commitment than more conventional service audits and evaluations. This can outstrip practitioner capacity if a large number of projects have to be undertaken at once. There is a need to carefully select which projects should be completed swiftly under normal monitoring conditions and which could meaningfully benefit from a wider co-production approach. Early engagement is also key to the co-production process and practitioners should be aware of the need to fully participate and that there may be additional calls on their time to attend shared meetings to establish efficient ways of working acceptable to all parties. The co-produced projects should also be seen as part of the mainstream work of the department and not a separate endeavour. Without this understanding it can be difficult to prioritise the total workload of the practitioner.

Imbalances in the time spent on a project can cause true co-production to collapse with one former partner taking on the lion share of responsibility for the project. The likelihood of this can be affected by a number of drivers. These may include other calls on time, prior experience and skills, as well as relative seniority. There is a risk therefore that a project can suddenly require a much larger share of an individual's time if it is to continue.

There are therefore strong benefits to an organisation promoting a co-production model between researchers and practitioners. There are additional benefits for the practitioner as an individual too as the research skills gained, reflecting a wider training than would normally be available, are transferable to new projects and can form the basis of further advancement.

In the broader sense of co-production, that of a relationship between service provider and user, which pulls together the knowledge, skills and resources of both groups with the aim of developing efficient, sustainable and acceptable responses to issues, also serves to reduce inequities by changing the balance of power from a top-down hierarchical professional to recipient arrangement to one of partnership. Following this model provides a fairer and more robust way of affecting change within communities or with individuals.

Co-production also has a pivotal part to play in the creation of acceptable and innovative public health interventions. In this context the co-production may be between service provider and user. This relationship is again based upon mutual trust and promotes the sharing of ideas; both in what needs to be prioritised for intervention and which interventions would be acceptable to the target population.

In "Commission on the Future Delivery of Public Services" (Christie, 2011), Dr Christie highlights the need for effective services to be designed in partnership with people and communities rather than in a top-down fashion to suit providers and commissioners. When delivered as part of an asset-based approach this will allow collaboration to promote the creation of efficient services that while being more person centred will also work sustainably. Co-production has been used at several levels, including redesign of health and social care services. This approach moves beyond only gaining the views of focus groups or undertaking formal consultation around already developed proposals but includes a range of stakeholders, for example at the programme board level.

Recently a new diabetes prevention framework has been published in Scotland (Scottish Government, 2018). Some early adopter NHS Boards have formed diabetes prevention partnerships to design and implement evidence based interventions acceptable to their communities. In doing so data has been gathered and analysed to develop health needs assessments, to measure the impact of services currently being used and perform gap analyses. Involving members of the community and service users in generating this information as well as on the strategic board responsible along with service providers, budget holders, health and physical activity professionals allows for deeper insights into what people see as being important issues, what may be done to better support the population's health, how this should be delivered and the ways in which messages and information should best be communicated. This form of collective working allows barriers and facilitators to be fully articulated by both professional and lay groups. It is therefore possible to minimise the effects of barriers and maximise the utility of any investment.

For example, group work may be promoted after members of patient groups express a need for peer support. The delivery times and sites of interventions may also be altered to meet local need. From a public health practitioner's point of view this information and consequent adjustment of plans is invaluable in delivering efficient, equitable, acceptable and sustainable programmes. Additionally this co-production approach may make it easier for the community to take ownership of activities undertaken.

In essence, co-production can deliver better outcomes for those involved; be it practitioner, researcher or service user. The approach can be integrated into co-commissioning, co-design of pathways, services or research questions or facilitate working in partnership with third sector groups and therefore promote the involvement of interested groups or indeed the wider community. In some sense it is listening to people with additional and specific experience and incorporating this into the planning or development process. However, true co-production moves beyond this to true partnership working and is therefore of importance to the public health practitioner as it is a tool for identifying the best tool for the job and the best way of delivering it. In doing so the practitioner must be aware that all relevant stakeholders are represented equitably so as not to bias outcomes.

Underpinning the co-production approach are the values of mutuality and respect (Stephens et al. 2008; Scottish Co-Production Network, 2015b). Recognition that different parties have expertise and providing a vehicle to access it is a powerful way of tackling inequalities. There may be some trepidation felt by practitioners in this move away from top down creation of services and pathways. This may be compounded by where the system traditionally puts accountability. It is therefore important to note the value to the practitioner in recognising within policy guidelines. An example of good practice in this is the current Scottish experience as a number of legal Acts, such as The Public Bodies (Joint Working) (Scotland) Act 2014, which amongst its principles highlights the need to make integrated services that are person centred and take into account the needs of service users whilst being led locally through community engagement; the person centred Children and Young People (Scotland) Act 2014; The Social Care (Self-directed Support) (Scotland) Act 2013, which seeks to move the locus of control from the state to a reciprocal position, and others that touch on the approach (Scottish Co-Production Network, 2015a).

Co-production of services or research is one element of an assets based approach to public health and salutogenesis. A further benefit to the public health practitioner in co-producing research with academics is the possible contributions to the literature, both in terms of the individual project findings and indeed the co-production approach itself. This serves to demonstrate the impact of the work itself, which is immediately useful to the practitioner, and also makes the distilled information more widely available. If the project itself has been co-produced with stakeholders this allows another route of dissemination of findings and provides an additional benefit to the researchers in having a diverse audience to talk with.

In summary, co-production is a useful approach to both research and more broadly in service design and delivery. From the public health practitioner's point of view it allows access to expertise that may not normally be available. This may be in terms of academic analytic and evaluative skills or in providing expert patient or service user insight into need and how that can best be served. Furthermore, through following a co-production approach, public health practitioners are likely to acquire additional skills that may be deployed on subsequent projects. Ultimately, this from of asset-based approach is likely to be useful in constructing more efficient, robust, effective and acceptable answers to public health problems.

Five top tips

- Be clear about the purpose of the project. The different parties within the co-production group may have different agendas and will certainly have different pressures on them. It is important therefore to have a clear idea from the outset what the group seeks to achieve and how success will be measured. This should be formed in early group discussions.
- Avoid 'mission creep'. It is understandable that those involved in a co-produced project will want to get the best from it and maximise their outcomes. A researcher may become interested in answering a new question arising from the data or a practitioner may want an additional programme element added or tested, for example. Where there is resource to address additional emergent priorities this is, of course, a positive and the synergy of skills within the group may allow for these to be addressed efficiently. However, these additional tasks should be agreed by the group and should take into account the initial purpose of the project as previously agreed.
- Gain agreement on realistic timelines and milestones. Public health practitioners and researchers will tend to have previously worked to different timescales. It is therefore important to establish how much time and focus to give different priorities. It is also important to establish the additional time needed to set up a research project when compared with a perhaps more familiar service review or audit. The time it takes to prepare documents and go through a research ethics committee can be significant and may not be part of a practitioner's normal working practice. It is therefore useful to not only form a timeline of these milestones early on but to establish what is in and out of scope for the various parties and what should be prioritised.
- Keep good lines of communication open. This underpins the previous points. It is important to have regular and inclusive meetings to stay on track and to raise any issues. If possible it is worth embedding staff, at least for part of the time, in the host organisation (e.g. a researcher in a local authority or NHS Board and a practitioner in a university setting). In practice this may be easier for some individuals than others. If a researcher is working on several projects with the same public health team it may be possible for them to dedicate some time to working in that team. This shortens lines of communication and allows for quick discussions to be had; however, as noted above, the group should be careful to guard against 'mission creep'. Similarly, it would be beneficial for practitioners to gain insight to the workings of a research team.
- Be aware of local priorities. By bringing together different groups we also bring together those groups priorities and politics. Furthermore, there is

the new dimension of how these interact to take into account. Again, having clearly agreed objectives will help with this, as will clear terms of reference and governance routes. To fully engage with the co-production process it is important that mutual respect is maintained at all times.

References

Christie, C. (2011). *Commission on the future delivery of public services.* [online]. Available at: https://www.gov.scot/binaries/content/documents/govscot/publica tions/publication/2011/06/commission-future-delivery-public-services/documents/ 0118638-pdf/0118638-pdf/govscot%3Adocument [Accessed 05/04/2019].

Scottish Government (2018). *A healthier future: type 2 Diabetes prevention, early detection and intervention: framework.* [online]. Available at: https://www.gov.scot/p ublications/healthier-future-framework-prevention-early-detection-early-interven tion-type-2/ [Accessed 05/04/2019].

Scottish Co-production Network (2015a). *Self management: Why co-production is central.* [online] Available at: http://www.coproductionscotland.org.uk/resources/ resource-case-studies/self-management-why-co-production-is-central/ [Accessed 05/ 04/2019].

Scottish Co-production Network (2015b). *Co-production in Scotland – a policy over-view.* [online] Available at: http://www.coproductionscotland.org.uk/resources/co-p roduction-in-scotland-a-policy-overview/ [Accessed 05/04/2019]

Stephens, L., Ryan-Collins, J. and Boyle, D. (2008). *Co-production a manifesto for growing the core economy.* [online] New Economics Foundation. Available at: https:// neweconomics.org/2008/07/co-production [Accessed 05/04/2019].

4 Working with schools to develop complex interventions for public health improvement

Jeremy Segrott and Joan Roberts

Introduction

In this chapter we explore the ways in which researchers can work collaboratively with schools to develop complex interventions designed to improve public health. We begin by summarising the importance of young people's health as a focus for this work, and the importance of schools as a setting for health improvement. We then turn our attention to the increasing emphasis now being placed on working collaboratively with schools to co-produce new health improvement interventions. Drawing on Wight et al.'s (2016) framework for intervention development – 6SQUID – we consider how this co-production can contribute to intervention development at four critical stages: defining the problem to be addressed by the intervention; which aspects of the problem are most amenable to change; defining and describing the change mechanisms that will achieve the intervention's key goals; and the formulation of implementation systems and strategies. We also examine how members of a school community can be involved in shaping the aims, design and conduct of evaluation studies that accompany intervention development. The final part of the chapter reflects on some of the key challenges that researchers face when seeking to co-produce interventions and possible strategies for overcoming these.

Children and young people's health as a public health priority

Promoting the health of children and young people is a key public health priority in the UK and many other countries around the world (Currie et al. 2009; Laski et al. 2015). A range of factors shape children and young people's health, spanning individual attitudes through family and peer networks to broad social and structural determinants. The environments in which young people live, and the health behaviours which they develop during childhood and adolescence, have been shown to shape long-term health outcomes (e.g. Metzler et al. 2017; Nurius et al. 2016). For instance, aspects of family environments may act as protective factors against later substance misuse (Segrott et al. 2015), whilst dietary habits formed during the early years can track through into adulthood (e.g. Garcia et al. 2014). Focusing on young people, adolescence is a period of transition accompanied by complex physical and psychological changes (Patton et al. 2016), and a range of external stressors including peer networks, and academic work and assessment. There are significant concerns regarding current levels of mental health problems among young people, and the best ways to address this (Gunnell et al. 2018; Patel et al. 2017).

Schools and the health and wellbeing of children and young people

Schools play an important role in shaping the health and wellbeing of children and young people. In various forms, health education has formed a part of the school curriculum for many decades and a central way in which to teach knowledge regarding health behaviours such as (un)healthy eating, substance misuse and mental health. Whilst classroom-based approaches to health promotion remain important, in recent years there has been a move to expand understanding of how schools shape the health of young people, school staff and others who interact with them through adoption of a Health Promoting School approach (sometimes referred to as a whole school approach) (Langford et al. 2017). This recognises that alongside tuition in the classroom, the school environment (social and physical) shapes health, and that connections between schools and families and the wider community are also important. It is also widely recognised that there are important relationships between young people's health and education (Durlak et al. 2011; Langford et al. 2017) – e.g. pupils who are happy and feel connected to school are more likely to achieve their full academic potential. Whilst schools have therefore traditionally been seen as spaces of education (and outside the remit of health policy and interventions) there is now recognition that schools influence young people's wellbeing, and that efforts to improve young people's health and wellbeing may have beneficial effects for educational engagement and attainment (Murphy et al. 2018). Schools are thus increasingly an important site for and target of health improvement interventions.

Researchers in the field of public health have accordingly looked for opportunities to develop and evaluate interventions in school settings – many of which take a whole school approach, linking classroom activities, changes to school environments (e.g. preventing bullying, modifying aspects of food provision) and strengthening connections between schools and parents/carers. Part of a more general recognition that many of the key influences on young people's health and settings for addressing them lie outside the healthcare system (Viner et al. 2012), school-based approaches to health promotion bring public health practitioners and researchers into an environment concerned primarily with educational instruction (Murphy et al. 2018), and one mainly assessed by its ability to do so.

Working with schools

Recognition of schools as a key setting for health improvement interventions has been an important step forward. But, in turn, it raises a series of questions concerning what the targets of change should be, which kinds of interventions are needed, and how they should be implemented. Perhaps too often intervention developers have been guilty of developing a new intervention (on say promoting healthy eating) without working collaboratively with schools or the multiple groups of individuals within them (staff, parents, other carers and children themselves). Whilst such interventions may draw upon academic theories concerning behaviour change processes, they have frequently failed to achieve their intended effects. As Kok et al. (2012) argue, traditionally a 'linear' approach to evidence-based practice has been adopted. Interventions have been seen as 'fixed entities' that remain the same as they are implemented in different contexts, with deviations from the standardised intervention seen as problematic.

It is now recognised that whilst interventions may be based on 'good science' and sound theory, they may fail to generate their desired effects because they do not achieve 'fit' or 'congruence' with the local context into which they are introduced (Murphy et al. 2018). Sometimes this concerns the chosen focus of the intervention (and how it aligns or not with a school's priorities), its relevance to the nature of the issue as it occurs within a school (a classroom-based intervention will not directly address aspects of the dining hall which influence pupils' diets) or challenges in implementing the necessary activities (it is not feasible to deliver it as intended or there is not the commitment to do so). Insights from studies of implementation have taught us that the key to an intervention's long-term sustainability is whether it is valued by those asked to deliver and support it, and if it is therefore integrated and embedded within an organisation's 'everyday business' (May, 2013).

In public health as a whole there has been a strong move for academics to work in partnership with those outside academia when developing and evaluating new interventions, partly in order to address the problems addressed above. Thus, it is now common to see academics work with practitioners and policy makers from the outset when designing new research studies. Involving the public in the development and evaluation of interventions has also become an important aspect of what we do. Inclusion of such groups indicates a willingness to value different experiences and views, and to treat those of members of the public (for instance) as being of equal value to those of academics. Another key driver for policy maker and public involvement is that it can improve the quality of interventions. It may help us to optimise the fit between intervention and the context (in this case schools) into which it is being introduced. Interventions developed in partnership with those asked to deliver – and receive them, may be better at identifying which mechanisms are most likely address a particular problem, which intervention activities have meaning and value, and optimal strategies for implementing them.

These issues become all the more important as the *type* of intervention we develop evolves. A whole school approach is likely to be concerned with making changes to aspects of school systems (norms, routines, structures, relationships) and not simply using the school as a place to reach large numbers of pupils. The need for whole school interventions to fit with and have meaning with local context is therefore even more pronounced, and critical in determining whether they are sustained over time (Murphy et al. 2018). Many of these principles have been captured within the work of Stokols et al. (2013) on Transdisciplinary Action Research (TDAR). Drawing on the principals of action research, TDAR seeks to identify problems and generate solutions by bringing together collaborations that stretch horizontally (across multiple disciplines and linking academics with policy makers and communities), vertically (e.g. national level policy with local organisations), and across sectors (e.g. linking activities across what are often siloed policy areas) (Hawkins et al. 2017). And there is a general move to conceptualise interventions as interacting with and drawing on aspects of the context into which they are delivered. As Kok et al. (2012) argue, we need to see interventions as comprising elements both of the original designer, and elements of the context in which they operate (e.g. funding, support networks).

Working with different members of school communities (pupils, staff and parents/carers) also has an important role to play in the design and conduct of research evaluations. It can help inform the research questions and aims we generate for studies, for instance, and help us make sense of what our findings mean. It is now widely recognised – both by researchers and funders, that when done effectively, public involvement can improve the quality of the research we conduct and help maximise the extent to which it achieves its potential impacts. We know too that involvement of the public, policy makers and practitioners has most impact when it is built into a study from the start and integrated into all stages of a project plan.

Working with schools at key stages in the intervention development process

Recent work by Wight et al. (2016) notes the paucity of guidance for researchers on how to develop new interventions, particularly for those interventions not primarily focused on multi-level or system-based approaches. They set out a useful six-step framework (6SQUID) for public health intervention development. In the sections below we consider how co-production work with schools might form an important part of the first four stages of the framework (stages 5 and 6 concern intervention testing and initial assessment of effectiveness and so are not covered here).

Stage 1: defining and understanding the problem and its causes

Wight, et al. suggest that the starting point for intervention development is to clarify and define the problem to be addressed. This involves working with stakeholders and examining the existing literature to identify how the identified problem may be distributed across social groups and place, and the key causes which underlie it.

A research team may start out with a clear idea of the problem they wish to address via a school-based intervention and there may be support for the scale of problem and its potential causes in the literature. Working with schools at this early stage can generate important new insights. Different groups (e.g. teachers, young people) may place differing emphasis on the importance of the problem identified by the researchers. Young people for example may identify other issues within the school environment which they feel have greater importance than the problem as originally defined by the researchers. For instance, whilst researchers may have identified excessive screen time as an important influence on sleep routines and other aspects of health, young people may be more concerned with aspects of peer relationships (and pressure) that take place via electronic devices. Discussions with schools at this point can therefore help shape researchers' thinking to respond to the needs of different groups, and help align new interventions with these needs from an early stage. They can also help clarify how different groups within the school understand a particular public health issue and its key causes. For instance, there are potentially many different factors that shape the diets and eating behaviours of children. An intervention that is focused on changing individual young people's attitudes may be misplaced if pupils themselves identify other factors which shape their diet, such as school food environments, the (in)ability to control what food is eaten or purchased at home, or the influence of peer networks. School staff may have valuable perspectives on how pupils' diets affect learning in the classroom, and the barriers to making changes to the school food environment.

A key point therefore is that working with schools can generate new perspectives that may not have been identified in the scientific literature or researchers' initial discussions (de Andrade et al. 2015), and help to more closely align the resulting intervention with the needs of schools, and the key factors driving a particular public health issue. For example, Hawkins, et al. (2018) built co-production with multiple groups into the development of a new school-based intervention to prevent substance misuse. Consultation with young people helped to identify which drugs were used most commonly by their age group (and therefore which might be included in the intervention), including some which had not been covered by previous research studies.

In our work on the development of an intervention to link secondary schools and families we have consulted with young people, school staff and parents/carers to explore their experiences and views from the outset. Through this work we have sought to understand whether these groups see family-school connections as important (and if so why), the challenges which they face in building these connections, and whether they would support the idea of developing an intervention to address them. This initial work identified broad support among young people, schools and parents/carers for developing these connections and highlighted some of the key barriers to doing so. These perspectives were particularly valuable given the significant gaps in the literature on health improvement interventions linking schools and families.

Stage 2: selecting which contextual factors should be targeted by the intervention

Wight, et al. (2016) suggest that the second stage of intervention development should be to "Clarify which causal or contextual factors are malleable and have greatest scope for change". Schools themselves can provide valuable insights into the extent to which aspects of a health issue (and how it operates within a school system) may be most amenable to change, and aspects which it may be impracticable or challenging to modify. Discussions with schools at this point can also reveal where support may lie for action. Such support is often linked to the extent to which an intervention aligns with the needs and priorities of schools, both in terms of how they view their role, and also the direction of regional or national policies.

There are various ways in which these kinds of discussions can be held with schools. Turning again to the authors' current work on the development of a new intervention to develop links between schools and families, our early engagement with schools has involved group-based discussions with young people and teachers and one-to-one consultation with parents/carers. We have asked these different groups about the existing links between schools and families, and whether (and if so why and for whom) they think these may be helpful. We have also asked them what kinds of new connections they would like to see in the future, and how they might benefit different groups. These discussions have helped us understand how different groups within the school conceptualise the issue we are interested in, how developing a new intervention might address their needs, and where we might begin to focus our attention. Our consultation with young people for instance identified that as they became more independent during secondary school they continued to value parental input around learning (particularly linked to time and stress management) and that for some issues parents fulfilled an important 'advocacy' role when issues needed to be discussed with school staff. For schools themselves we have looked at where the proposed intervention might have fit with national policy, and in particular how it might enable schools to demonstrate their achievements in these areas. A key example is the way in which links with and support for families now features strongly within the schools inspection framework in Wales.

Stage 3: identifying how to 'bring about change'

Once the key causal factors to be addressed have been established the next stage is to identify what Wight, et al. describe as the intervention's 'causal mechanisms' – that is, how the intervention will impact on the problem being addressed. They suggest that a useful part of this work is to develop a logic model – which shows diagrammatically how an intervention is designed to work, linking activities with short-term outcomes, which in turn may trigger long term outcomes. The authors suggest that whilst use of formal theories is a crucial part of this task, it is also important to consult with stakeholders.

School staff, pupils and parents will frequently have useful input and insights to contribute to an early version of an intervention logic model. Consultation with different groups within schools can identify which of the hypothesised outcomes have most importance or relevance. This can be helpful in identifying likely levels of support within schools, and ways in which the intervention can be framed in ways that maximise its relevance for individuals who will deliver and receive it. It is also valuable to understand whether interventions and their intended activities and goals are seen as acceptable to different parts of the community – particularly in relation to sensitive or potentially stigmatising topics.

A crucial insight that members of a school community can share with researchers is the extent to which the theory of change outlined in a logic model is likely to operate in the intended way within a school context in general, and in more specific school settings. For example, proposed intervention activities may function in different ways to those intended, or it may be that they are unlikely to be sufficiently intense or sustained long enough to deliver the intended changes. There are also many examples in the literature of evaluations of interventions, which when implemented have created unintended (and unexpected) harmful effects. For example, Sorhaindo et al. (2016) describe how the Young People's Development Programme – a targeted school-based intervention that aimed to prevent teenage pregnancy – actually increased pregnancy rates. Some of the young people who received the intervention described negative experiences in relation to the intervention, including feelings of being stigmatised and labelled. Where young people are involved in the design of interventions at an early stage they may be able to identify such issues, which can then be used to modify intervention design, framing and activities.

A key point here is that the move towards whole school approaches to health promotion means that increasingly interventions are working simultaneously at different levels (individual, peer groups, school environment and policy, links with parents and families) rather than just targeting individual behaviours and awareness. As Murphy et al. (2018) argue, such whole school interventions are often concerned with trying to change aspects of the school system – and they therefore need to adapt to and become adopted by school communities themselves. Paying attention to the ways in which an intervention's core goals can be integrated within and embedded within a school system is therefore of pertinence for these types of interventions.

Stage 4: delivering the change mechanisms

It is important to consider how the proposed intervention will be delivered – both in terms of its format, who will deliver it (school staff, external agencies), and how implementation will be organised (who will coordinate delivery and pay the necessary delivery costs?). A key issue that researchers need to bear in mind during this stage of intervention development (in addition to the earlier phases) is the extent to which an intervention helps address schools' own goals, and how intervention activities can become integrated within schools and sustained over time. Those interventions that have poor fit with schools' goals and priorities are unlikely be implemented well (if at all) and may be discarded once the involvement of a research team ceases. Asking teachers to take on burdensome tasks as part of an intervention is unlikely to be feasible. Likewise, interventions that cost significant sums of money may be much harder to sustain over time than those which can be implemented as part of existing roles and responsibilities. Delivery of interventions by external providers – whilst reducing the burden on staff – may be a barrier to integration within schools, especially if the intervention takes the format of a one-off educational session for pupils. These concerns shaped our own approach to refining a primary school-based intervention with a family component designed to prevent alcohol misuse. Through input from teachers and other education practitioners, the intervention was designed to align closely with, and help schools achieve some of their existing goals so that rather than being a separate, external task, it could become incorporated within the school system. The classroom work which formed part of the intervention was designed to address directly the National Curriculum whilst the family component could fit within schools' existing work around family engagement. In line with this approach, schools themselves were responsible for delivery of the intervention, with the aim that this not only reduced the cost and complexity of arranging external facilitation, but also helped ensure that it became part of schools' ongoing work (Rothwell & Segrott, 2011; Segrott, et al. 2015).

Evaluation of interventions

Although this chapter is focused primarily on co-production of interventions it is helpful to consider how researchers engaged in this task are often also simultaneously running a research study as they develop their intervention. There are important ways in which members of school communities can be involved in shaping aspects of the research element of these studies. Working with students and teachers at the outset of a research project (and ideally at the grant development stage) can be invaluable in refining the understanding of the problem to be addressed (as discussed above) and the key research questions which the study should consider. Ideally, input from schools should be built into all of the main stages of a research project. In our own work we have benefitted greatly, for instance, from working with groups of pupils in schools to consult on key aspects of our study. This has included seeking their advice on recruitment strategies, the design and content of information sheets and consent forms, and the design, clarity and acceptability of data collection tools. In our feasibility study examining a primary school-based alcohol misuse prevention intervention, we asked groups of pupils to read through and provide critical feedback on our proposed questionnaires. Their feedback included, but extended well beyond, issues of clarity of meaning and presentation. For instance, they provided new insights for us on how different kinds of questions might be viewed as sensitive. Whilst we initially anticipated that questions on substance use would potentially be the most problematic aspect of the questionnaire, they suggested that the section asking about family and household composition was an area that other children their age might find sensitive, or at least uncomfortable to answer. As a result we were able to revise these questions to increase their acceptability and to avoid inadvertently suggesting that only certain household compositions were 'normal'.

Key challenges in working with schools

Identifying adequate resources

As we have argued above, co-production activities have an important role to play throughout the different stages of intervention development (and as part of the broader research study within which it sits). Working with schools from the beginning can help to maximise the extent to which they can shape the intervention and build meaningful long-term relationships. Paradoxically though, funding for such involvement (at a point where it may make the biggest impact) is limited. There are relatively few funding schemes for instance which cover the costs of working with schools during the preparation of research funding applications, but at a point when important decisions may be being made about the framing of the intervention's goals or design. The danger here is that important insights are missed in the early stages of intervention development or that at a later stage of an intervention's development school community members identify issues which it is more difficult or too late to address.

The introduction of funding schemes specifically focused on intervention *development* (as opposed to *evaluation* studies) such as the UK Medical Research Council's Public Health Intervention Development scheme are extremely helpful in providing a source of funding for researchers to work with schools during the initial stages of intervention development. In our own research centre – DECIPHer, we have also been fortunate to be able to access support from specialist public involvement staff and a school health research network, which help facilitate access to schools. We have also been able to use the Public Involvement infrastructure, which is funded by our research centre – particularly its young people's advisory group (ALPHA). Whilst not school-based, this group has enabled us to explore the kinds of questions we have posed above in relation to school-based interventions with young people.

Building capacity and capability

When school staff or students are asked to work with researchers to co-produce interventions it is important to identify whether these groups may need – or indeed want to receive, training and new skills. For example, teachers may have little or no formal research training, and are unlikely to be familiar with the concept of intervention logic models or have experience in critically appraising academic papers (though they bring important knowledge and experience to these tasks).

Similar issues arise when working with children and young people. It is important to ensure that discussions, concepts and information provided are age appropriate and clear and accessible. Equally it should be remembered that children – from quite an early age, can reflect on and express sophisticated opinions on a range of complex topics. In our experience it is perfectly possible to discuss complex ideas (e.g. consent, factors shaping health behaviours, the functioning of family relationships) with children in primary schools, if this done in an approachable, sensitive and age appropriate manner.

Co-production also requires various skills and competencies on the part of researchers. Training in what may be variously referred to as public involvement, public engagement, or co-production is a relatively recent phenomenon. Increasingly, researchers are likely to wish to – and often be required to – undertake some form of public involvement as part of their studies, but may not have extensive training or experience in undertaking it. Whilst some aspects of traditional research training may be helpful, co-production also requires other skills (such as framing research concepts for members of the public, or how best to work with schools), which may not be covered. To some extent these revolve around the ability to translate theoretical, conceptual or statistical information into a form which is understandable for a lay (or non-academic) audience.

A number of authors have noted that there is still relatively little methodological guidance on intervention development (e.g. Wight et al. 2016; Hawkins et al. 2017). This general comment applies also to the work of co-producing interventions and research studies with schools. It is an issue that needs addressing, particularly since the field in general is moving towards interventions that seek to interact with, and shape schools as complex systems. As Murphy, et al. (2018) note, where interventions seek to modify school systems it is important that they have 'congruence' with the existing systems. They argue that "there has been a failure to integrate academic, policy, practice and public communities to co-produce school health improvement research and build in processes to understand intervention congruence with existing systems and structures, and hence their sustainability". Co-production therefore arguably has a heightened role and importance as we move towards developing system-level interventions, which depends on achieving congruence with the organisations (such as schools) into which they introduced.

Working in schools

Whilst schools are often an enjoyable and supportive environment to work in, there are also several challenges that working in this setting can generate. Schools – by their very nature – are busy and pressured organisations with many calls upon their time and energy. It can be difficult to identify and recruit schools that are willing to find time for pupils and/or staff to contribute to providing input during the intervention development process (and possibly beyond) – potentially through multiple meetings or discussion groups as the project progresses through subsequent stages. Often researchers are keen to engage with schools in different contexts so as to include school communities with contrasting socio-economic and cultural backgrounds. Thus recruitment is more involved than simply identifying a single school that is keen to be involved in research or with which a researcher has an existing connection. The need to think about reaching different groups is also pertinent once a researcher has obtained permission to work with a school. It may often be difficult, for instance, to engage large numbers of parents/carers, or to establish how representative those that do express an interest may be of the wider population. These issues are important because it is helpful to know to what extent an intervention is likely to reach and meet the needs of parents/carers (for instance) from a range of different backgrounds, and these viewpoints need to inform initial intervention development.

Conclusion

The health and wellbeing of children and young people is a key priority in the field of Public Health. Schools are an important setting in which to develop, implement and evaluate health improvement interventions. A whole school approach emphasises that multiple aspects of schools shape young people's health, including education in the classroom, the school environment, and connections with parents/carers and the wider community. In this chapter we have highlighted some of the important ways in which co-production with schools can contribute to the development of school-based interventions, including those which adopt a whole school approach. It is now widely recognised that researchers (and others) cannot develop new interventions and then simply expect schools to deliver them. Co-production of new interventions with school staff, pupils and parents/carers offers several critical advantages. Foremost among these is the fact that interventions which are produced collaboratively with schools are likely to be better interventions (though research on this question is limited). At a broad level, co-production can help develop interventions which have better fit with the context into which they are introduced, meet the needs of those they are designed to help, and are more likely to be sustained. Specifically, we have explored how co-production can help at different stages of the intervention development process, including framing the problem to be addressed, identifying which factors may be amenable to change, building a theory of change, and forming effective strategies for implementation. Working collaboratively with schools signals that researchers value the voices and experiences of non-academics – and that they have an important part to play in shaping the interventions which researchers wish to develop.

We have also identified some of the challenges to co-production in schools, including recruitment, funding, and building skills – both for researchers and members of school communities. Current efforts to develop research infrastructures that support co-production – such as funding schemes for intervention development, specialist practitioners that can link researchers and schools, and opportunities for training, are important. These steps will help not only to provide practical support and improve the quality of the co-production that we do, but also signal that it has a valuable role to play in optimising the quality and impact of the interventions we develop.

Five top tips

- Build co-production into all stages of the intervention development and evaluation process – start as early as possible.
- Co-production can help shape: definition of the 'problem' to be addressed; the key factors which influence it; how to bring about change in these factors; the best methods for intervention delivery.
- Explore the views of different groups within schools who may have contrasting needs or perspectives (teachers, other school staff, pupils, parents/carers).
- Use co-production to help identify ways in which an intervention can achieve 'fit' and 'alignment' with school contexts. This can help bring about change in school systems, and sustain and embed intervention activities over the longer term.
- Identify and respond to the training and skill development needs of researchers, school staff, young people and parents/carers when co-producing an intervention.

References

Currie, C., Zanotti, C., Morgan, A., Currie, D., de Looze, M., Roberts, C., Samdal, O., Smith, O.R.F., and Barnekow, V. (2009). *Social determinants of health and well-being among young people: Health Behaviour in School-Aged Children (HBSC) study – International Report from the 2009/2010 Survey.* Copenhagen: WHO Regional Office for Europe.

de Andrade, M., Angus, K., Hastings, G. (2015) 'Teenage perceptions of electronic cigarettes in Scottish tobacco-education school interventions: Co-production and innovative engagement through a pop-up radio project'. *Perspectives in Public Health*, 136(5), 288–293.

Durlak, J., Weissberg, R., Dymnicki, A., Taylor, R., Schellinger, K. (2011) 'The impact of enhancing students' social and emotional learning: A meta-analysis of school-based universal interventions'. *Child Development*, 82(1), 405–432.

Garcia, A., Vargas, E., Lam, P., Shennan, D., Smith, F. and Parrett, A. (2014) 'Evaluation of a cooking skills programme in parents of young children – a longitudinal study'. *Public Health Nutrition*, 17(5), 1013–1021.

Gunnell, D., Kidger, J. and Elvidge, H. (2018) 'Adolescent mental health in crisis'. *BMJ*, 361, k2608.

Hawkins, J., Madden, K., Fletcher, A., Midgley, L., Grant, A., Cox, G., Moore, L., Campbell, R., Murphy, S., Bonell, C., and White, J. (2017) Development of a framework for the co-production and prototyping of public health interventions. *BMC Public Health*, 17(1), article number: 689. (doi:10.1186/s12889-017-4695-8).

Kok, M., Vaandrager, L., Bal, R., Schuit, J. (2012) 'Practitioner opinions on health promotion interventions that work: Opening the "black box" of a linear evidence-based approach'. *Social Science and Medicine*, 74(5), 715–723.

Langford, R., Bonell, C., Komro, K., Murphy, S., Magnus, D., Waters, E., Gibbs, L., and Campbell, R. (2017) 'The Health promoting schools framework: Known unknowns and an agenda for future research'. *Health Education & Behavior*, 44(3), 463–475.

Laski, L. (on behalf of the Expert Consultative Group for Every Woman Every Child on Adolescent Health). (2015) 'Realising the health and wellbeing of adolescents'. *BMJ*, 351, h4119.

May, C. (2013) 'Towards a general theory of implementation'. *Implementation Science*, 8, 18.

Metzler, M., Merrick, M., Klevens, J., Ports, K., Ford, D. (2017) 'Adverse childhood experiences and life opportunities: Shifting the narrative'. *Children and Youth Services Review*, 72, 141–149.

Murphy, S., Littlecott, H., Hewitt, G., MacDonald, S., Roberts, J., Bishop, J., Roberts, C., Thurston, R., Bishop, A., Moore, L., and Moore, G. (2018) 'A Transdisciplinary Complex Adaptive Systems (T-CAS) approach to developing a national school-based culture of prevention for health improvement: the School Health Research Network (SHRN) in Wales'. *Prevention Science* (published online).

Nurius, P., Green, S., Logan-Greene, P., Longhi, D. and Song, C. (2016) 'Stress pathways to health inequalities: Embedding ACEs within social and behavioral contexts'. *International Public Health Journal*, 8(2): 241–256.

Patel, V., Flisher, A., Hetrick, S. and McGorry, P. (2007) 'Mental health of young people: a global public-health challenge'. *The Lancet*, 369(9569): 1302–1313.

Patton, G., Sawyer, S., Santelli, J., Ross, D., Afifi, R., Allen, N., Arora, M., Azzopardi, P., Baldwin, W., Bonell, C., Kakuma, R., Kennedy, E., Mahon, J., McGovern, T., Mokdad, A., Patel, V., Petroni, S., Reavley, N., Taiwo, K., Waldfogel, J., Wickremarthne, D., Barroso, C., Bhutta, Z., Fatusi, A., Mattoo, A., Diers, J., Fang, J., Ferguson, J., Ssewamala, F., and Viner, R. (2016) 'Our future: a Lancet commission on adolescent health and wellbeing'. *The Lancet Commissions*, 387(10036), 2423–2478.

Rothwell, H. and Segrott, J. (2011) 'Preventing alcohol misuse in young people aged 9–11 years through promoting family communication: an exploratory evaluation of the Kids, Adults Together (KAT) Programme'. *BMC Public Health*, 11(1), 810.

Segrott, J., Rothwell, H., Pignatelli, I., Playle, R., Hewitt, G., Huang, C., Murphy, S., Hickman, M. and Moore, L. (2015) 'Exploratory trial of a school-based alcohol prevention intervention with a family component: Implications for implementation'. *Health Education*, 116(4), 410–431.

Sorhaindo, A., Bonell, C., Fletcher, A., Jessiman, P., Keogh, P. and Mitchell, K. (2016) 'Being targeted: Young women's experience of being identified for a teenage pregnancy prevention programme'. *Journal of Adolescence*, 49, 181–190.

Stokols, D., Hall, K. and Vogel, A. (2013) 'Transdisciplinary public health: Definitions, core characteristics, and strategies for success'. In D. Haire-Joshu and T.D. McBride (eds), *Transdisciplinary public health: Research, methods, and practice*, Edition. Hoboken, NJ: Jossey-Bass, pp. 3–30.

Viner, R., Ozer, E., Denny, S., Marmot, M., Resnick, M., Fatusi, A. and Currie, C. (2012) 'Adolescence and the social determinants of health'. *The Lancet*, 379, 1641–1652.

Wight, D., Wimbush, E., Jepson, R. and Doi, L. (2016) 'Six steps in quality intervention development (6SQuID)'. *Journal of Epidemiology and Community Health*, 70(5), 520–525.

5 Pupils, teachers and academics working together on a research project examining how students and teachers feel about the new GCSEs

Michael Chay Hayden, Gillian Waller, Abbey Hodgson, Scott Brown, Sean Harris, Katie Miller, Daniel Barber, Lewis Hudson and Dorothy Newbury-Birch

Overview

This chapter will present the research methods and the findings of Team Alpha and Norham Together (TALeNT), a research project that involved academics working collaboratively with staff and students from a secondary school in the North East of England. Team TALeNT was formed in summer 2016, and consisted of both academics from Teesside University and students and the Assistant Head Teacher from Norham High School in North Shields. The project initially set out to introduce the students to research, and the process involved in conducting a research project, but it also acted as a platform for students to gain new skills and build confidence in preparation for higher education and differing career paths (Bynner and Parsons 2002). Evidence shows that statistically significant positive relationships exist between the number of employer contacts, such as careers talks or work experience, that a young person experiences in school, between the ages of 14 and 19 years, and their reported confidence at 19–24 years in progression towards ultimate career goals; the likelihood of whether (at 19–24 years) they are NEET or non-NEET; and their earnings if salaried (Bynner and Parsons 2002).

Introduction

Norham High School is a smaller than average-sized secondary school based in the North East of England, with 323 registered students in the academic year 2016/2017 (GOV.UK 2017). The majority of students are of White British heritage, with only 2.5% not having English as a first language, compared to the national average of 16% (GOV.UK 2017). The total percentage of students with a statement of special education needs (SEN) is nearly twice the national average at 7.1%, compared with 4.3% (GOV.UK 2017). In addition,

62% of Norham's students receive free school meals, compared with the national average of 29%, highlighting the deprivation of the local community (GOV.UK 2017). When the young people involved in this project were asked about people's perceptions of Norham High School, they were quick to talk about it having a "bad reputation" and students there "not always having chances or opportunities". Nevertheless, they also talked about the "differing personalities of students", and Norham remains vibrant with a plethora of teachers who are wholly committed to furthering the education of the students.

Professor Newbury-Birch is an ex-pupil of the school and was invited to go back into the school in the spring of 2016 to discuss her journey from leaving Norham High School to becoming a Professor. As a result of this an innovative project was proposed in summer 2016 between Norham High School and the Alcohol and Public Health Research Team (Team Alpha) at Teesside University. The project involved research staff working with six students, across their journey from Year 9 to Year 11, to develop and carry out a research project that was largely led by the students.

Meetings

In the first instance, the research group was set up and regular meetings were held at Norham High School with both the students (MCH, AH, SB, KM, DB and LH), the research staff (DNB and GW) and a senior member of staff from Norham (SH). Meetings occurred every other month, after school and had a clear objective at the start of each session, with students being responsible for taking notes. Following a group discussion, the research group was named Team TALeNT, with TALeNT being an acronym of Team Alpha and Norham Together. The name was significant as it highlighted the importance of adopting a co-production approach of working together to undertake the research project (Verschuere et al. 2012).

In order to ensure the project was as successful as possible, the first meeting set out to discuss and formalise the terms of reference for Team TALeNT going forward. One of the key points was ensuring that although the students would view the adults as leaders, that everyone in the group was equal with everyone being able to have a say on the direction of the project and the meetings. This was extended to include only using first names to address each other instead of using titles and surnames (Dr, Prof, Mr or Ms), and this was agreed as an important way to achieve equality within the group.

Another of the key terms was that the decisions at all stages would be discussed and agreed. It was put forward that all members should attend at least 75% of the scheduled meetings to stay involved in Team TALeNT. However, and importantly, if an individual fell below that amount they would not be automatically ejected from the group without discussing why they hadn't been able to come and a decision would be made within the group whether they should stay involved. As it was, all Team TALeNT members were able to attend the proposed 75% of meetings.

Research topic

The first, full-day Team TALeNT meeting was designed to discuss the potential areas of research in order to reach a consensus within the group around a definitive research topic. The day at Norham High School was spent employing different techniques to explore all of the research areas that were put forward. The young people were first asked to reflect upon the areas that were most important to them and that interested them the most. An important structuring approach was using mind-maps to display figuratively the different areas of interest. A comprehensive discussion ensued that discussed the potential of approximately 50 different research areas. The topics discussed were largely heterogenous and ranged from military history; conflict resolution; the supernatural and stress amongst students. With support from the research staff, the young people were then able to make a list of the most popular areas in order to narrow down the research options. A series of cuts to the list was made, with voting occurring within the group at each stage. This was repeated until only two options remained which were conflict resolution within the school and the effect of the changes to the old GCSE's on both young people and teachers.

The final decision was made by the students themselves with the changes to the GCSEs being the most popular choice. By providing the students with the final decision on the research area, it ensured that the young people felt they were key players for the decision making for the topic and would therefore feel a sense of ownership of the project from the beginning.

In order to provide some background to the chosen research topic, the changes to the GCSE exams will be briefly discussed. Following a reconstruction within the 2016–2017 academic year, the traditional GCSE exams were modified resulting in a new grading system and an increased level of content (Long 2016; GOV.UK 2017; Barrance and Elwood 2018). The changes were proposed as a way in which to achieve improved recognition of the differing abilities of pupils within secondary schools, and specifically recognising pupils of higher ability by introducing more demanding content (Long 2016; GOV.UK 2017; Barrance and Elwood 2018).

The biggest change made to the GCSEs, was around the existing grading system. Previously GCSE exams were graded using A*to G grades; whereas the newly implemented system employs numerical grades (Long 2016; GOV. UK 2017; Barrance and Elwood 2018). For each academic subject, pupils now seek to obtain a grade between 1 to 9, with grade 9 being the highest achievable grade (Long 2016; GOV.UK 2017; Barrance and Elwood 2018). This has caused confusion with both teaching staff and young people, as it has not always been clear how each alphabetical grade translates to a numerical grade. Therefore, this was thought to be a fundamental area to explore within this research project. Further changes were made to the GCSE course structures, and their academic contents underwent modifications in order to further challenge pupils, and to eliminate the coursework aspects, in favour of examinations (Long 2016; GOV.UK 2017; Barrance and Elwood 2018).

Aim

After deciding upon a research area, it was important to propose an overall aim for the research project. This was assisted by the research staff explaining to the young people the importance of having an aim in order to direct the research. This led to the collective development of this aim: "to explore the recent changes to the GCSE system, focusing on how the changes will impact both staff and students".

Research methods

The research that was undertaken consisted of semi-structured interviews with an opportune sample of students in Years 9 and 10 and school staff.

In order to sufficiently explore the aim of the project, different research methods were discussed and explained within a Team TALeNT meeting. It was proposed that to explore the different perceptions and views around the GCSE changes, it was most appropriate to conduct qualitative, one-to-one interviews with Norham High School staff and students. The one-to-one interview type identified as being the most suitable was the semi-structured interview, as they allow a flexible approach to be adopted (Green and Thorogood 2011; Bryman 2015). This meant the young people did not have to rigidly adhere to the interview schedule and could probe the participants on any interesting responses that came out (Green and Thorogood 2011, Bryman 2015).

The young people were given the task to develop the required information sheets and consent forms. With the help of the research staff, they were successfully able to develop an information sheet for the school staff and the students, and a consent form to be completed prior to the interview commencement.

Recruitment of the interview participants was first initiated in the school summer term of 2017. In order to be able to recruit the young people to take part in an interview, letters were sent to the parents or caregivers of Norham students in Years 9 and 10, informing them of the research with an information sheet. In addition, an opt-out form was included, in order for parents to be able to opt their child out of the research if they wished.

The interviews took place over two days in the school during school hours in July 2017. The Team TALeNT students conducted all of the semi-structured interviews and were responsible for identifying students and staff to take part, with the support of the university researchers. A member of staff (DNB,

GW or SH) sat in on all of the interviews to support the young person and to ensure they were comfortable and able to understand and ask all of the questions appropriately.

The sampling method was opportunistic as on the days of the interviews, any young people in Years 9 and 10 or school staff, who were able to assent or consent to take part, were invited to take part in one-to-one interview (Suri 2011). Prior to the interview commencement, interview participants were given the information sheet to read through and were reminded that their participation was voluntary and that they were free to withdraw at any time. Participants were also assured that any identifying information would be removed and their responses would remain confidential, unless a safeguarding issue arose that would need to be reported to the school staff. Following this, all participants were instructed to complete an assent (young people) or a consent (school staff) form to take part (Miller et al. 2004). All interviews were then recorded using a Dictaphone to aid the transcription process.

During discussions within the Team TALeNT sessions, a semi-structured interview was developed by the young people, with help from the university staff (Green and Thorogood 2011). The schedule guided the interviewers to ask participants a series of questions to ascertain their views on what they thought about the new GCSE system. For students, these included questions around preparedness, workload, stress and support from the school, friends and families. For staff the questions were around preparedness, workload, stress as well as whether students had required or asked for more support in relation to the new GCSE's.

Training

As previously mentioned, the young people were responsible for conducting all of the interviews with staff and students. As the young people had no previous experience of conducting research, it was important to ensure that they received adequate training so they felt confident and possessed the skills and knowledge to undertake the research activities. Therefore, training was provided by the research staff at various stages of the project.

In order to prepare for conducting interviews, the research staff went through the basics and the important things to remember whilst conducting an interview. The young people then had a go at asking interview questions, in a role play in front of the group, whilst the research staff acted as teachers. This was an important way of developing the interview skills required and built the young people's confidence. Following the training, the Team TALeNT group discussed important points to remember and areas to improve on which aided the learning process.

If, following training, a young person still didn't feel comfortable undertaking an interview, they were encouraged to take part in the coordination of the research and the recruitment of the participants, to ensure that they still played an active role in the data collection process.

Data analysis

All of the interviews were audio recorded, transcribed verbatim and anonymised before being analysed thematically (Ritchie and Spencer 1994; Braun and Clarke 2006). Applied thematic analysis is a phenomenological approach to qualitative analysis that focuses on the individual experiences of participants (Ritchie and Spencer 1994; Braun and Clarke 2006). Analysis begins with line-by-line coding of transcripts with similar codes being grouped together into themes and sub-themes. An inductive approach was used when coding the transcripts as no existing theory was used to facilitate the coding, in order to ensure the coding process was accessible for the young people (Ritchie and Spencer 1994; Braun and Clarke 2006). A Team TALeNT data analysis meeting was set up, which involved each transcript being coded in groups by the young people, with help from the university staff. Using coloured pens to highlight and code similar responses, overarching themes were able to be identified. These themes were discussed further and agreed by all members of the group.

Results of research – young people

Seventeen interviews were carried out with young people. Following the coding and the analysis of the transcripts within the group, four main themes were identified from the interviews around the changes to the GCSEs. These were: Confidence; Confusion around how GCSEs are scored; Support from school staff and Workload. These areas have been unpacked in more detail below using quotes to illustrate the main findings.

Confidence

A key theme that emerged from the young people's interview data was around confidence. This was widely reflected upon and generally the changes made to the GCSEs, have left students feeling less confident, due to the increased workload and most importantly not knowing what to expect from the new exams.

> Some of them I feel like I'm not very good at, or some I'm not very confident that I'm going to pass, with a good grade.
>
> (Pupil 8)

> I think it might make it more difficult for our year group to achieve the grades that we want, like, previous years have had, good grades because the GCSEs have been similar, for them all the way through school, but with us, we've had to change, from, what we were taught in Year 7, to 9 and in Year 10, to change what we're doing now.
>
> (Pupil 17)

However, in contrast some participants did feel they were confident they would get their target grades, but only if they put in enough work.

> I mean, I'm worried about all tests, but I'm pretty confident if I work hard, I'll get good grades.
>
> (Pupil 6)

Therefore, although the levels of confidence did appear variable across the young people interviewed, it was apparent that a large proportion of young people were experiencing low levels of confidence.

Confusion around how GCSEs are scored

A second richly populated theme was the feeling of confusion, specifically around the new GCSE grading system. There was a great feeling of confusion around what to expect and what young people needed to do to achieve their desired target grades.

> well I understood the old GCSEs, and the new GCSEs, I'm a bit confused on, what grade means what.
>
> (Pupil 3)

> Cos we've been in the, GCSEs for a while, and all of a sudden, they turn around and say no, you've got to get a different grade now.
>
> (Pupil 5)

In addition, when participants were asked what grades they needed to pass, some students referred to the old grading system (A*–G), and when asked if they knew the corresponding numerical grade (1–9), they were often unable to quantify them.

> Yeah, minimum C Grade.
>
> (Pupil 7)

> A 'C' isn't it? Or, I dunno.
>
> (Pupil 15)

This indicated that generally young people did not feel confident translating the new grades, they struggled to understand the new numerical system and were unsure on what grade they should be aiming for.

Workload

One of the biggest changes made to the GCSEs was the increase in content and it was apparent across the board that the young people interviewed agreed about the increased amount of work they now needed to do to pass. In addition, they frequently reflected upon the content appearing more challenging and the need to do more work to keep up with the material.

> It'll be a lot harder and we'll have to study more.
>
> (Pupil 13)

Interview participants also talked about needing to do more than they used to and having to get used to the transition of needing to work hard and revise more outside of school hours.

> I end up doing a lot more revising than I used to, usually like, maybe about, five, six hours a week or something.
>
> (Pupil 7)

Support from school

Finally, on the whole, the young people interviewed were positive about the support they were receiving from their secondary school around their GCSEs. More specifically, young people could talk about particular teachers and the techniques that they found the most helpful and supportive.

> Just helping us a lot, and then giving us, more support than, others, like not just individually, I mean (.) making us understand things more.
>
> (Pupil 3)

> Yeah, just like giving wer, a good amount of work, and asking if we need any help.
>
> (Pupil 8)

Specific strategies that were favoured were ones that helped young people learn how to revise and memorise the increased content of the new exams. Additionally, young people preferred teachers who were active and dynamic, and could make learning the increased content fun and engaging.

> He, when he teaches, he's like, he's active about it, he makes it interesting, which makes us do more, because I'm interested in it.
>
> (Pupil 16)

A small minority of the students interviewed were not happy with the support they were receiving from the school, and felt that some teachers could do more to help them better navigate the changes to the GCSEs.

> Most of them are, but some, just don't, don't feel like they care.
>
> (Pupil 2)

Therefore, although the majority of young people were positive about the support they were receiving within school, specific subjects and members of staff were responsible for some young people feeling unsupported.

Results – teaching staff

Four interviews were conducted with teaching staff. The main themes that came out of these interviews were around Anxiety about results or pupil performance; Differing learning and teaching mechanisms; and Collegiate working. Again, these areas have been unpacked in more detail below using direct quotes to illustrate the main findings.

Anxiety about results performance

Similarly, to the young people interviews, all of the staff interview participants reflected upon possessing a degree of nervousness or anxiety about their pupils achieving their target grades. This was largely due to a plethora of different reasons, but a common factor was thought to be a result of the increase in academic content.

> I think there is some level of anxiety and I think some element of frustration. A number of staff, have sort of said, that they're concerned with how much sheer content there is.
>
> (Teacher 2)

This anxiety also extended to include teachers themselves feeling unsure about what a student would need to do to achieve a specific grade, as the new grade boundaries and marking criteria were not known.

> We don't quite know what the grade boundaries are, so we don't know what is going to be required to get to that grade 4 or 5.
>
> (Teacher 1)

Not knowing the grade boundaries left staff feeling anxious, as they felt less confident in reassuring the students around performance.

Differing learning and teaching mechanisms

Adapting to the new GCSEs and the increased amount of content has also resulted in school staff needing to modify and adapt their learning and teaching mechanisms. This was an area widely reflected upon within the staff interviews as they have had to explore new techniques of supporting students.

> I know some staff are a bit concerned because they are having to adapt, the way they teach because of it.
>
> (Teacher 2)

Specific examples of this that were cited included building in quizzes to track progress and helping the young people to develop their revision skills.

> build in all those regular little quizzes and checks, particularly around vocabulary and key facts, so to help build a student's confidence, that they are coping with it, and that they do understand the stuff, because teaching a GCSE over 3 years is a long time for students to be working on something.
>
> (Teacher 1)

> I'm having to try and teach more revision techniques over time. How we, train our brain in to learning some of the information.
>
> (Teacher 2)

Collegiate working

There was a strong theme of collegiate working apparent within the school staff interviews. The school staff frequently reflected upon the importance of sharing good practice, working together, and supporting other members of staff to ensure the transition over to the new GCSEs was as smooth as possible.

> I think teachers need time to work together and talk with other teachers, in other schools because, other people always have really good ideas that you just haven't thought of, and that makes life easier.
>
> (Teacher 1)

A specific example of support that was discussed was both in-house and external training. Teacher 4 talked about the importance of being able to receive training that could be filtered down to other members of staff within the school.

> Continuing to have support and the flexibility to go out, continuing to go on exam CPD sessions.
>
> (Teacher 4)

Therefore, staff working together within the school and extending to share good practice across other secondary schools, was seen as a facilitator of adapting to the changes in the new GCSE system.

Discussion

Following the completion of the research project it was clear how the new changes to the GCSEs had impacted both the school staff and the students (Long 2016; GOV.UK 2017, Barrance and Elwood 2018). It will be important for school staff to reflect upon these results in order to ensure that secondary school pupils are adequately supported when undertaking their GCSEs. The results may also prove useful to young people undertaking their GCSEs or those about to embark on them, by ensuring they do not underestimate the workload and the challenging content.

The running theme across both sets of participants (students and staff) was the idea of uncertainty and feeling anxious about the young people being able to achieve their target grades (Putwain et al. 2016). As the new GCSEs become more established and common place within the school system, these feelings have the potential to ameliorate, but it was recognised as important to try new teaching techniques and strategies to maximise the current practice. In addition, the feelings of anxiety directly link with the confusion around not knowing which numerical grades equate to which alphabetical grades, but again over time, the transition to the numerical grades will become increasingly normalised.

The results of the interviews also highlighted the importance of supporting both school staff and the students with the GCSE changes. Staff support appeared to be the most beneficial when staff shared good practice, working together and learning from others (Darling-Hammond 2003, Brandon and Charlton 2011). Young people support was most effective when teachers had dynamic learning styles and could help with revision. This finding is consistent with the work of Muijs and Reynolds, which agrees that dynamic and interactive learning are key components of effective teaching (Muijs and Reynolds 2017).

Although the aim of Team TALeNT was to conduct a piece of research with young people driving the project, it was most important to discuss and reflect upon the benefits to both the young people and staff involved with the project. This chapter will conclude by discussing the learning gained from this and presents the top tips of conducting a co-production research project within a school setting.

Learning

In regards to the learning obtained from conducting academic research collaboratively within a school setting (Hewitt et al. 2018), it was important to ensure all of the young people felt confident and supported when undertaking the research activities. As previously discussed, some of the young people in Team TALeNT did not feel comfortable conducting an interview. This meant they could get involved in other activities, such as organising the interviews, which played to their individual strengths. The key learning from this is ensuring that tasks are allocated appropriately and being clear about the expectations or requirements of each task.

A question at the end of the interview schedule also sought to explore the views of both staff and students on young people carrying out research in a school setting. The responses to this were overwhelmingly positive with both staff and students agreeing it "developed young people's skills", "gave young people a voice" and "was a fantastic opportunity".

Being a part of Team TALeNT also proved significant benefits to the university researchers as it gave them an opportunity to further develop their skills of working with and engaging young people, whilst developing their teaching and training skills. When undertaking the brainstorming of initial research ideas, it also provided an opportunity to identify the most important and topical areas for young people.

The five top tips that have been learnt from conducting co-production research within a school setting will be used to ensure that the next cycle of Team TALeNT, will be as successful and rewarding for the new cohort of students and staff.

Top five tips to school-based co-production research

- Ensure that research staff have the correct checks in place to be allowed to work in the school.
- Students should be involved from the inception to the dissemination of the research project. In addition, allocating the research tasks appropriately, by considering an individual's strengths is important, so that all members of the group feel comfortable.
- Good communication is imperative. Being clear from the outset of the expectations and requirements of students and staff makes a project run more smoothly.
- Training and support is important to build both skills and confidence, but it should be pitched at an appropriate and accessible level for young people.
- Ensuring that everyone is treated equally and that everyone is able to get their opinion across – reinforcing that no question is a stupid question!

References

Barrance, R. and J. Elwood (2018). "National assessment policy reform 14–16 and its consequences for young people: student views and experiences of GCSE reform in Northern Ireland and Wales." *Assessment in Education: Principles, Policy & Practice*: 1–20.

Brandon, T. and J. Charlton (2011). "The lessons learned from developing an inclusive learning and teaching community of practice." *International Journal of Inclusive Education* 15(1): 165–178.

Braun, V. and V. Clarke (2006). "Using thematic analysis in psychology." *Qualitative Research Psychology* 3(2): 77–101.

Bryman, A. (2015). *Social Research Methods*. Oxford: Oxford University Press.

Bynner, J. and S. Parsons (2002). "Social exclusion and the transition from school to work: The case of young people not in education, employment, or training (NEET)." *Journal of Vocational Behavior* 60(2): 289–309.

Darling-Hammond, L. (2003). "Keeping good teachers: Why it matters, what leaders can do." *Educational Leadership* 60(8): 6–13.

GOV.UK. (2017). *Find and Compare Schools in England: Norham High School.* Retrieved from https://www.compare-school-performance.service.gov.uk/school/108628?tab=absence-and-pupil-population.

GOV.UK. (2017). *Get the Facts: GCSE Reform.* Retrieved from https://www.gov.uk/government/publications/get-the-facts-gcse-and-a-level-reform/get-the-facts-gcse-reform.

Green, J. and N. Thorogood (2011). *Qualitative Methods for Health Research,* New York: Sage Publishing.

Hewitt, G., J. Roberts, A. Fletcher, G. Moore and S. Murphy (2018). "Improving young people's health and well-being through a school health research network: Reflections on school–researcher engagement at the national level." *Research for All* 2(1): 16–33.

Long, R. (2016). *GCSE, AS and A level Reform (England).* House of Commons Briefing Paper, Number 06962, 5 January 2016, from https://dera.ioe.ac.uk/25291/2/SN06962_Redacted.pdf.

Mann, A. (2012). *It's Who You Meet: Why Employer Contacts at School Make a Difference to the Employment Prospects of Young Adults.* London: *Education and Employers.*

Miller, V. A., D. Drotar and E. Kodish (2004). "Children's competence for assent and consent: a review of empirical findings." *Ethics & Behavior* 14(3): 255–295.

Muijs, D. and D. Reynolds (2017). *Effective Teaching: Evidence and Practice,* London: Sage.

Putwain, D. W., A. L. Daly, S. Chamberlain and S. Sadreddini (2016). "'Sink or swim': buoyancy and coping in the cognitive test anxiety–academic performance relationship." *Educational Psychology* 36(10): 1807–1825.

Ritchie, J. and L. Spencer (1994). Qualitative data analysis for applied policy research. In A. Bryman and R. Burgess (eds), *Analysing Qualitative Data.* London: Routledge.

Suri, H. (2011). "Purposeful sampling in qualitative research synthesis." *Qualitative Research Journal* 11(2): 63–75.

Verschuere, B., T. Brandsen and V. Pestoff (2012). "Co-production: The state of the art in research and the future agenda." *Voluntas: International Journal of Voluntary and Nonprofit Organizations* 23(4): 1083–1101.

6 Public health practitioners and academics working together to evaluation a mental health youth awareness programme

Natalie Connor, Michelle Baldwin, Gill O'Neill, Gillian Waller and Dorothy Newbury-Birch

What is the Youth Aware Mental Health Programme (YAM)?

The Saving and Empowering Young Lives in Europe study (SEYLE) was a cluster randomised control trial (RCT) that compared the efficacy of school-based preventative interventions of suicidal behaviours (Wasserman et al. 2015). Three interventions and a control group were compared. One of these interventions, the Youth Aware of Mental Health Programme (YAM), was associated with a significant reduction of incident suicide attempts and severe suicidal ideation compared with the control group. YAM has been designed for use in the classroom as a universal evidence-based mental health promotion programme for 14–16-year-olds. The aim of the programme is to help students explore their experiences of mental health using role play, as well as reflect on previous actions and reactions. In addition, pupils are provided with a resource guide of local health resources and different organisations who work with young people in the community.

YAM is a structured programme that is delivered by trained facilitators in the school setting. Facilitators attend a training programme delivered by a team from the National Centre for Suicide Research and Prevention of Mental Ill-Health (NASP) at the Karolinska Institutet and Columbia University. This team were commissioned by Durham County Council to deliver the YAM training to staff in County Durham. The staff trained included a mix of school, resilience and educational psychology nurses. The program typically lasts for five weeks, with an introductory lesson followed by four distinct lessons, each of which lasted an hour and explored various scenarios linked to mental health through role play.

The SEYLE study, carried out in nine countries and across five continents, found YAM to be effective at improving several mental health outcomes, such as reducing depression and reducing suicide attempts (Wasserman et al. 2015). Furthermore, the YAM programme was shown to encourage understanding between pupils, encourage peer support and allow pupils to get to know each other better, helping them to understand that they were not alone with their problems and thus they were more likely to seek help when needed.

YAM also helped adolescents who had existing mental health problems as the programme included facilitations of clinical evaluation and help (Wasserman et al. 2015).

Why is YAM useful?

Approximately 615 million people worldwide, both adults and children, have issues with mental health (Chisholm et al. 2016). At least one in four people will experience a mental health issue at some point in their lives (McManus et al. 2009). More recently, a YouGov online poll revealed that 51% of adults who had felt stressed in 2018 reported feeling depressed, with 61% having feelings of anxiety (Mental Health Foundation; 2018).

Mental health problems were reported to cost the UK economy an estimated £70–100 billion in 2015 (Mental Health Foundation 2016). Yet public spending on mental health is focussed almost entirely on coping with crisis, rather than investing in prevention (Mental Health Foundation 2016). Mental illness and self-injury account for 23% of the UK's disease burden, compared to 16% for cancer and 16% for cardiovascular disease (WHO (2008) 'The Global Burden of Disease, 2004 update').Yet despite this, mental illness received only 13% of NHS health expenditure (Centre for Economic Performance 2012).

The mental health of young people is a global concern (Sawyer et al. 2012). Research indicates that one in ten children aged 5–16 years has a mental health problem, and half of those with lifetime mental health problems first experience symptoms by the age of 14, (Sawyer et al. 2012; Green et al. 2005) and three-quarters before their mid-20s (Kessler and Wang 2007). The Prince's Trust carried out their annual Macquarie Youth Index in 2017, which showed that the wellbeing of young people under the age of 25 has dropped to its lowest level in their survey since the study was launched in 2009 (The Prince's Trust Macquarie Youth Index 2017). In total, 48% of the 2215 young people surveyed experienced problems that prevented them focusing on their studies, and nearly half of those who had experienced a problem did not talk to anyone about their situation. Of those who had experienced a problem, 32% did not know who they could talk to. A total of 78% felt that there was stigma attached to mental health issues which was a barrier to them discussing their problems (The Prince's Trust Macquarie Youth Index 2017). Furthermore, one in 12 children and young people deliberately self-harm, and approximately 40,000 cases of self-harm by children and young people result in hospitalisation each year (Young Minds and The Cello Group 2012). Therefore, early intervention for youth mental health problems is likely to result in long-term health and societal gains (Sawyer et al. 2012; McGorry et al. 2007; Schaffalitzky et al. 2015).

Those who describe themselves as having positive mental health and wellbeing are reported to have a range of better outcomes across all ages and backgrounds. These include improved physical health and life expectancy, better educational achievement, increased skills, reduced health risk behaviours such as smoking and alcohol misuse, reduced risk of mental health problems and suicide, improved employment rates and productivity, reduced anti-social behaviour and criminality, and higher levels of social interaction and participation.

Why an implementation evaluation?

This evaluation was one of a number of co-production evaluations undertaken between Teesside University and Durham County Council. An implementation evaluation was agreed upon, as the SEYLE RCT had already proven the effectiveness of YAM; however, the feasibility and acceptability of such a programme in County Durham was untested. In order to evaluate the implementation of this programme process data was collated and pupils, school staff and delivery staff were invited to take part in focus groups to discuss barriers and facilitators to the successful implementation of the programme. The primary aim of this evaluation was to determine whether YAM was a feasible delivery model that was sustainable within the school environment in County Durham. Seven schools took part in the year one pilot, and seven schools in year two (two schools from year one, and five new schools). Six of these schools were involved with the evaluation.

YAM is currently being evaluated by the Department of Education in a large-scale randomised control trial, which will span over 200 schools in England. DNB is a member of the steering group for the study. The RCT follows on from a report by the Institute for Public Policy Research, which said all secondary schools needed access to a mental health professional on site, at least one day a week, to combat anxiety and depression. Two other interventions will be evaluated alongside YAM, a Canadian model called 'The Guide' and a lighter-touch preventative programme. However, this data will not be available until at least 2020.

Major learnings from practitioners

This section will describe what the co-ordinators and staff who delivered the YAM programme have learnt within the first two years of the YAM roll-out across County Durham, as well as the key learning points from the academic team using co-production methods.

2017 Delivery staff findings

Delivery staff focus groups took part in year one and again in year two of YAM implementation. All staff who had completed the YAM training programme in 2017 were invited to take part in a focus group Four focus groups were held: two just after the initial roll out of YAM had begun, and two following the completion of at least one YAM programme per staff member. The focus groups were analysed using applied thematic analysis (Joffe and

Yardley 2012). Four major themes emerged from the analysis of focus groups: initial training and understanding of YAM; benefits of YAM for staff and students; barriers to schools engaging with YAM; and suggested changes to improve delivery of YAM. The first theme, initial training and understanding of YAM, was not evident in the second round of focus groups in 2018. However, some key findings from this theme are summarised below, and may be useful for other local authorities in England who wish to roll out YAM to secondary schools.

It was felt that it was crucial for staff members who signed up to become YAM instructors to have a good understanding of what YAM entailed. The training course was described as fantastic and of value, but quite intense, therefore staff needed to be prepared. In addition, staff needed to be passionate about what YAM aims to achieve with young people. One of the added benefits of training was the course helped to develop relationships internally within DCC, with partnerships and key networks built. A substantial amount of preparation time was required prior to starting any delivery, to ensure that all administration tasks were covered, booklets were prepared with local information, and workloads managed. Allowing sufficient time to ensure the logistics of delivery were correct was seen by delivery staff as important in easing the pressure of first time delivery. It was suggested that having slightly more practice time before delivery commenced would be beneficial.

Moving forward, staff felt that it was important that school group sizes were smaller, i.e. 15. This would help with managing challenging behaviour, but also would allow delivery staff additional time with pupils to build relationships and trust. Room set-ups with flexibility in moving chairs and tables would facilitate better sessions. Also, schools that had flexibility in how long sessions lasted (between 45 minutes and an hour) found it beneficial in engaging different groups. Finally, a need to invest in training additional staff and further training for current staff in areas such as behaviour management was articulated. It was also recognised that additional time spent planning future delivery in year two should focus on creating an equal workload across delivery staff. As a result of this early work, changes were made to how the YAM program would run in year two.

2018 findings

In year two of the roll-out, all delivery staff were invited to take part in a second phase of focus groups. Three major themes emerged from the analysis of focus groups: benefits of YAM for staff and students; barriers to schools engaging with YAM; and suggested changes to improve delivery of YAM.

Benefits of YAM for staff and students; developing relationships and networks

Becoming involved with the YAM programme was not only seen as part of the day job, it was seen as something that had enabled staff to develop new skills that they could take away and use in other parts of their role. As well as up-skilling, staff felt that the expansion of their colleague network, and liaising with teams who would normally work in different areas had improved efficiency in certain areas. The introduction of training up 'helpers' to support YAM trained instructors was seen as a positive development, based on feedback from delivery staff after year one. The increased staff numbers has allowed for a greater consistency with who delivers sessions together. This, in turn, has enabled relationships and dynamics to develop. A number of helpers have gone on to become trained YAM instructors, and this pathway from helper to instructor has helped to ease earlier concerns from staff in year one, who weren't sure what to expect, even after a week of training:

> I think the training was very good but it's very difficult to imagine what it's going to be like when you're actually there delivering. It was beneficial, being a helper first because I was petrified, just the thought of it. Standing up and doing it regardless of training. Being a helper let me see what the sessions were like before having to take charge and lead.
>
> (Phase two – P1)

Pupil engagement and wider benefits of YAM

Following on from delivering the first round of YAM programmes, staff reported that they were really pleased with how some of the pupils had responded to the programme, and engaged with the sessions:

> Some of them (pupils) had clearly been thinking about it from one week to the next, already had ideas of what they wanted to cover in role plays.
>
> (Phase one – P3)

This finding was supported with data from second phase focus groups:

> It was the way that a number of children in every group had talked to us – they would say, this is what I'm struggling with and then we could sign post to other support. It makes it all worthwhile.
>
> (Phase two – P6)

Staff also commented in the different ways that pupils engaged, and even when it appeared that pupils weren't benefitting from the programme, something would happen to change that opinion:

> My one who came at the end on Thursday, on the last session, she's talked the whole way through, she's been disruptive ... she's failed to

engage ... yet at the end of session five, or I thought she had, yeah, she's come and she's like can we talk? You know I've been thinking about this, and what we've said in here, and I've thought wow!

(Phase one – P11)

You're right, if you can get even one child at the end of it that feels they can come forward, then it's worthwhile isn't it?

(Phase one – P9)

Delivery staff highlighted how they were growing in confidence to use novel ways to engage pupils, as YAM continued to be embedded, and that engagement was sometimes only evident towards the end of a programme:

The boys weren't engaging. It was when the world cup was on. One lad drew a flag so I asked him to write in the white bits what he had learnt from YAM and he did. Instead of saying you're not supposed to do that, it was manageable.

(Phase two – P15)

It was noted that the benefits extended beyond the interaction with an individual, and that the YAM programme was equipping the pupils with skills to then support their friends in the future if there was ever an issue. This perceived confidence to speak to their friends about mental health issues was seen as key to helping reduce isolation amongst young people, and YAM was empowering the pupils to have those mental health conversations. In addition, YAM was seen to provide another point of contact for those pupils who were most vulnerable. Whilst the long-term impact of YAM will hopefully empower young people to manage mental health issues in the best way they can, the short-term impact is simply having someone to talk to during a moment of crisis:

Barriers to schools engaging with YAM

A number of barriers to schools participating in the YAM pilot were highlighted throughout the focus groups by delivery staff. One of these barriers was school staff not feeling comfortable with being outside of the classroom when YAM sessions were being delivered. Even in schools that engaged with YAM, there was the suggestion that school staff were still entering the sessions. This can have a negative impact on how pupils engage with the programme:

One school we went into, they were struggling to hand the class over to us. The idea of YAM is that we're not teachers, on a couple of occasions I felt the class were settling in then the teacher would come in and sensed at times I wouldn't get as much from them.

(Phase two – P2)

Another potential barrier was the feeling that YAM would duplicate other programmes already running in particular schools. Some of these programmes, however, are not delivered across all schools in County Durham. This was supported by findings in school staff and pupil year two focus groups.

Delivery staff reported that a potential barrier to taking part in YAM was the fact that it is a very new programme, yet to be tested in England. This fear of the unknown, coupled with the sensitive nature of the topics covered in the programme may have stopped schools signing up:

> I think as well it's new. It's not happened anywhere else in England and it's ... some schools might be thinking, "Well if it doesn't work we'll be in the middle of this."
>
> (Phase one – P4)

Delivery staff felt that it was important that schools could see the value in embedding YAM into their school programmes. In addition to a fear of the unknown, there was also a sense of schools not signing up if particular teachers did not feel that mental health was an issue in their respective school, and that their pupils did not need YAM:

> That's still part of the issue, that a lot of the teachers don't see it (mental health) as a problem and we're trying to put it across that it's a universal programme, it's a preventative health promotional programme for all children as part of PHSE.
>
> (Phase one – P3)

The feedback from the school staff about the roll out of YAM was very positive, with teachers happy with how the pilot had progressed. However, the YAM delivery staff felt that there were a number of teething problems in year one which needed to be addressed to improve the programme. One of these involved the initial roll out of information, with some schools not being sure what YAM entailed. This was addressed with communication to schools, but one area that has emerged from the second wave of focus groups is the cascading of information about what YAM actually is from school staff to pupils:

> Some did it ... depends on the school. Some schools were good at communicating about what it is. Other came and said I have no idea why I'm here.
>
> (Phase two – P13)

Suggested changes to improve delivery of YAM

As mentioned previously, delivery staff felt that being a 'helper' before going through the Yam training to be an instructor was helpful, and could potentially be a pathway that is embedded for delivery staff. This would help to increase staff confidence before delivering, as well as ensure that staff are truly passionate about YAM before undertaking the training course:

> I was a helper before I was trainer and that's been a massive advantage. Instead of being freshly trained and going in and delivering, I had the experience and gained tips and knowledge. I would hate to think I was going in without being a helper. Spread it out; be a helper and then go in and deliver.
>
> (Phase two – P21)

Some delivery staff felt that it would be beneficial to have more understanding of each school's behaviour management policy before starting a YAM programme, so that there is an understanding of how to deal with issues before they actually arise. This could potentially link into the earlier suggestion from programme co-ordinators, about developing a delivery guide for YAM that is specific to County Durham.

An issue that was raised previously in phase one of the focus groups, was the difficulty in having sessions in different schools on different days of the week, especially when they were booked last minute. There have been changes to delivery to accommodate for this, such as an increase in staff members trained, and forward planning to try and create an efficient system for delivery, for example, delivering two programmes in one school in one afternoon. However, due to the co-ordinators trying to be as flexible as possible with schools, there were still occasions when the sessions were not consistent.

It was identified that further work was needed in communicating YAM and the role the programme played in improving resilience and wellbeing, amongst wider staff members of the school. Increased awareness from all staff members in a school that has signed up to YAM will improve the support mechanisms in place for pupils:

> The idea that wherever they are going to after they have had YAM the member of staff needs to know that they have just had YAM that would make sense. They need enough awareness to know where they've come from when they land in the class looking tearful. They need an idea of what is going on.
>
> (Phase two – P11)

There was also a suggestion from delivery staff to explore how programmes could be flexible in the future, to cover topics that a particular school felt were relevant but hadn't be covered. An example of this is one school in the second year of delivery requesting sessions on boys' mental health, and the stigma around males:

> At the end I asked them about in particular what we don't cover and what they would like to talk about and 2 of the 'popular' boys didn't say

it but wrote down on paper about talking about only boys and the stigma of boys.

(Phase two – P1)

I find that comes across a lot and talk a lot about that in groups – about how boys have to be macho and they never realised they don't have to be like that.

(Phase two – P3)

Finally, some delivery staff felt that YAM was appropriate for Year 9s, but that it should be introduced as a concept at a younger age so that pupils were aware of it in their school. There was also agreement that a follow-up session could take place in Years 10 and 11, which supported findings from the school staff and pupil perspective.

Summary: learning points from co-production

Co-production is seen as an approach where people, organisations and commissioners work together to share their skills and experience to design, deliver, monitor and evaluate services and projects. In this particular case study, evaluating the YAM programme by utilising a co-production approach was seen as vital, as trying to embed and drive forward the first YAM programme in England was untested.

Five top tips

- There is a considerable lead in time necessary for longer-term evaluations of programmes jointly produced by academics and public health practitioners. This may not be familiar to all stakeholders and so the time needed to go through the process of developing a protocol, gaining ethical approval, collecting necessary data and performing meaningful should be clearly articulated and agreed from the beginning. There should be an appreciation of the pressures to implement a programme quickly.
- With a shorter timeframe, pressure is on to collect data. In this evaluation, the early focus groups didn't give the true snapshot of how YAM was embedded, but were great for working through teething problems. When the programme hasn't been delivered by anyone else in the country, there is no one to go and ask and the pioneering nature of delivery staff should be recognised and commended. In this case, they have helped to shape the YAM programme, as they requested a 'Train the trainer' model from the YAM developers, and have also had an input into how training is now delivered. Good communication and feedback between parties is therefore key to improvement.

- Early focus groups have tremendous value, as the co-production method allows continuous feedback through the evaluation. Therefore services can be revised earlier in the process without the need to wait until the end of the evaluation before looking at recommendations.
- Individuals should be aware of the environment and context they are working in. This is true of both practitioners and academics. There is a need to be aware that political and structural pressures may differ between settings potentially having complex impacts upon working practices. This may include differences in practices between organisations but also the unexpected effects of larger change or interest from national bodies. In the context of YAM there was the opportunity to provide input to the Department of Education as they became interested in YAM and similar programmes.
- There is an enthusiasm and thirst for co-production that stems from a real desire to create services that are of value to the people who will use them. However, it is no easy task, with many opportunities to get things wrong. Nevertheless, if the necessary time is given to ensuring the right people are involved from the beginning, a robust protocol can be developed that can have room to be flexible to meet the varying demands of both practitioners and academics. This will give the best chance for the staff and partners who deliver services, as well as those who use them, to be allowed the opportunity to contribute their knowledge and experience towards improving the direction and quality of their service in the future.

References

Centre for Economic Performance. (2012) How Mental Illness Loses Out in the NHS. London: Centre for Economic Performance.

Chisholm, D., Sweeny, K., Sheehan, P., Rasmussen, B., Smit., F., Cuijpers, P., Saxena, S. (2016) Scaling-up treatment of depression and anxiety: a global return on investment analysis. *The Lancet Psychiatry*, 3, 5, 415–424

Green, H., McGinnity, A., Meltzer, H., Ford, T., and Goodman, R. (2005) *Mental Health of Children and Young People in Great Britain, 2004*. Basingstoke: Palgrave Macmillan.

Joffe, H. and Yardley, L. (2012), eds. *Content and Thematic Analysis. Research Methods for Clinical and Health Psychology*, ed. D.F. Marks and L. Yardley, Sage: London.

Kessler, R. and Wang, P. (2007). The descriptive epidemiology of commonly occurring mental disorders in the United States. *Annu Rev Public Health* 29, 115–129.

McGorry, P.D., Purcell, R., Hickie, I.B., and Jorm, A.F. (2007) Investing in youth mental health is a best buy *Med J Aust* 187: S5–7.

McManus, S., Meltzer, H., Brugha, T., Bebbington, and Jenkins, R. (2009) *Adult Psychiatric Morbidity in England, 2007: Results of a Household Survey*. Leeds: NHS Information Centre for Health and Social Care.

Mental Health Foundation (2016). *Research Strategy 2016–2020*. Retrieved from: https://www.mentalhealth.org.uk/sites/default/files/Research%20strategy%202016-2020.pdf

Mental Health Foundation (2018). *Results of the Mental Health Foundation's 2018 study.* Retrieved from: https://www.mentalhealth.org.uk/statistics/mental-health-sta tistics-stress

Sawyer, S.M., Afifi, RA, Bearinger, L.H., Blakemore, S.J., Dick, B., Ezeh, A.C., and Patton, G.C. (2012) Adolescence: A foundation for future health. *Lancet* 379: 1630–1640.

Schaffalitzky, E., Leahy, D., Armstrong, C., Gavin, B., Latham, L., McNicholas, F., Meagher, D., O'Connor, R., O'Toole, T., Smyth, B.P., and Cullen, W. (2015) Nobody really gets it: A qualitative exploration of youth mental health in deprived urban areas. *Early Interv Psychiatry* 9, 406–411.

Young Minds and The Cello Group (2012) *Talking Self-harm.* London: Young Minds and The Cello Group, October.

The Prince's Trust (2017) *Macquarie Youth Index*, available at: http://tinyurl.com/youth-index-20107

Wasserman, D., Hoven, C., Wasserman, C., Wall, M., Eisenberg, R., Hadlaczky, G., Kelleher, I., Sarchiapone, M., Apter, A., Balazs, J., Bobes, J., Brunner, R., Corcoran, P., Cosman, D., Guillemin, F., Haring, C., Iosue, M., Kaess, M., Kahn, J., Keeley, H., Musa, G., Nemes, B., Postuvan, V., Saiz, P., Reiter-Theil, S., Varnik, A. Varnik, P. and Carli, V. (2015). School-based suicide preventions programmes- the SEYLE cluster-randomised, control trial. *The Lancet*, 385, 9977, 1536–1544.

WHO (2008) 'The Global Burden of Disease, 2004 update'; 'No health without mental health: a cross-government mental health outcomes strategy for people of all ages – impact assessment', Department of Health, 2 February 2011 (para.1.17) www.gov. uk/government/uploads/system/uploads/attachment_data/file/213761/dh_124058.pdf

7 "It's not about telling people to eat better, stop smoking or get on the treadmill"

Mandy Cheetham, Sarah Gorman, Emma Gibson and Alice Wiseman

In the following chapter, we describe an example of a collaborative embedded research (ER) project, to develop a community-led, place-based approach to address childhood obesity. We draw on the perspectives of staff from the voluntary and community sector, local government and academia who were involved in the project.

Background and context

Gateshead Council have a track record of testing new approaches to public health challenges. The Director of Public Health could see the benefits of having an embedded researcher working on a childhood obesity project in an area facing significant health inequalities. In Gateshead at the time National Child Measurement Programme data (Gateshead Council JSNA 2018) showed that 23.2% of Year 6 children were classified as obese and 36% had excess weight (overweight and obese). Alice Wiseman (Gateshead Director of Public Health) commented:

> We are well aware that the burden of obesity is falling hardest on those children from low-income backgrounds. Obesity rates are highest for children from the most deprived areas and rates are rising. Children aged 5 from the poorest income groups are twice as likely to be obese compared to their most well-off counterparts and by age 11 they are three times as likely to be obese. Previous interventions have had limited success in reducing rates of obesity.

The Foresight report (Government Office for Science 2007) suggests that tackling obesity is complex, and the scale of the challenge requires action at an individual, community and societal level (Government Office for Science 2007). A 'place-based', community centred approach (South 2017) is a different way to develop local solutions that draw on all the resources in an area. This approach has the potential for people to take control of their health and wellbeing and allow them to influence the factors that underpin good health. Co-produced in partnership with local communities, the approach encompasses Gateshead's commitment to integrating evidence in to practice. As Alice acknowledged: "We knew we could not solve a complex problem with a linear solution".

Multi-agency partnership

The partnership involved Gateshead Council, Pattinson House, a community development organisation, and a researcher from Fuse, the Centre for Translational Research in Public Health (www.fuse.ac.uk).

Pattinson House was launched in 2015 by the charity Edberts House (http://www.edbertshouse.org/), and funded by the People's Health Trust. The project works to build a happier, healthier, friendlier community, and aims to reduce health inequalities by addressing the wider determinants of health. After a 12-month period of engagement, a community hub was created in the heart of an estate in Gateshead, facilitated by experienced community development staff and managed by a steering group of local residents.

Through the hub, community members are encouraged to build supportive relationships with one another, working together to identify key issues in their area and manage a budget to create activities and make their area an even better place to live. Within this context of well-established community development and relationships of trust, it was possible to host a thematically specific piece of research: the focus on obesity became a vehicle to test the underlying proposition that a community-led approach to a specific problem could lead to some innovative and sustainable change.

Embedded researcher

An embedded researcher based with the public health team, was invited to help understand what community-led interventions might be effective in tackling childhood obesity. ER involves a particular form of evidence co-production and use, which takes account of local context and stakeholder interests (Holmes et al. 2017; Rycroft-Malone 2014).

Embedded researchers have been defined as "either University based or employed, with the purpose of identifying and implementing a collaborative, jointly owned research agenda in a host organisation in a mutually beneficial relationship" (McGinity and Salakangas 2014: 3). Gateshead is an early adopter of the approach, which has been gaining interest in the UK as a way to create evidence-informed impact in service improvement (Marshall et al. 2016; Vindrola-Padros et al. 2017) and public health (Cheetham et al. 2017).

Meaningful engagement of communities in areas of socio-economic disadvantage is particularly important given recognition that they are often left out of research on obesity (Blacksher and Lovasi 2012). First-hand perspectives on health inequalities do not always inform public health research, policy or practice.

We hoped this study would offer local community members opportunities to identify and explore the issues they prioritised, whilst designing and participating in a range of activities. The process of co-producing and joint planning can be, in itself, health enhancing (Whitehead et al. 2016). The importance of creating the conditions for people to take control of their lives and places was highlighted by Marmot (2010):

> Autonomy, how much control you have over your life – and the opportunities for full social engagement and participation are crucial for health, wellbeing and longevity.
>
> (Marmot 2010: 2)

The ER approach was not without its critics, however. All three partner organisations were challenged about the value, methodology and potential risks of an ER project of this kind. Questions were raised about the wisdom of allowing a researcher open access to a community organisation without knowing what they might uncover. Others questioned the iterative nature of the research process, how outcomes would be measured, whether the researcher would become emotionally involved and lose the objectivity valued in some traditional academic quarters. There were also doubts about whether the research would be publishable in academic journals. There did not seem to be a lot of encouragement as we embarked on our *Fit for the Future* journey. Everyone seemed to be focussed on risk and what might go wrong, as Sarah Gorman, Chief Executive of Edberts House observed:

> I had only ever thought of the embedded research as a fantastic opportunity. An external pair of eyes on our work to help us articulate the value of what we are doing, plus the chance to identify our weaknesses and to try and develop. The presence of the researcher did not feel like an imposition or a 'spy in the camp' as people were suggesting!

Gateshead Council

ER was a relatively new way of working for Gateshead Council and some people had understandable concerns about reputational risk. It took persuasion by the Director of Public Health that this was the right approach to take. Other Councils have subsequently commented on how 'brave' and 'bold' the Council were in terms of managing the 'unknowns.'

Organisations that open themselves to the levels of scrutiny involved in this kind of insider research, take enormous risks. ER can reveal attitudes and behaviours that may not sit comfortably. Senior leaders in the organisations involved need to be willing to open themselves up to scrutiny, risk exposing vulnerabilities, both with staff, community members, and wider stakeholders, with whom information may be shared. The process can be threatening, and potentially cause long term damage to relationships, so must be handled with both sensitivity and bravery, whilst not shying away from potentially uncomfortable truths, as Sarah comments:

> The embedded researcher doesn't just see you on your good days. You can't put on a show! If they are with you for a whole year, they will really see you: your relationships, the way you do things, your values, so the research has real authenticity.

Shared values and non-judgemental attitudes and, most fundamentally, trust, were essential to make the project work:

> I knew that Alice and Mandy were both on a genuine journey of discovery – as were we. Our work is a complex adaptive process, and the research was absorbed into that, changing and enhancing our culture, allowing us to learn together. There was no fear of recrimination or blame if the project didn't live up to expectations – it was based on mutual trust and respect.
>
> (Sarah Gorman, Edberts House)

Where we started

At the beginning of the process, community members took part in organised conversations with the Director of Public Health, and further peer group conversations, as well as informal chats over lunch and activities, spending time with one another, staff and the researcher. They received training in creating power point presentations, and, supported by community development staff, formulated some initial ideas. They presented these ideas to the Director and a public health consultant in a lunchtime presentation – the first time that they had ever given a formal presentation. Sarah Gorman observed:

> Community members were really scared when they had to give the presentation – it wasn't something that they were used to doing, but particularly for one or two of them, it was a really significant moment in their personal development. One is now employed within the project: she grew so much in confidence, and really found her voice.

Each of the three partners recognised the mutually beneficial opportunities for connection that existed within the project, not just for people to get to know one another, but also to broker connections between local people and decision makers in the local area. Community members did not know that there was a Director of Public Health at the meeting, or what she did. Neither did they know what an embedded researcher was. Similarly, Alice and Mandy had not lived on the estate, and had not experienced the challenges faced by local people. Coming together to focus on the project with the shared experience of 'not knowing' changed the balance of power in the relationships. It challenged some of the potential barriers that can exist in traditional research projects. Instead of 'parachuting' into projects for a couple of man-ufactured focus groups, analysing and writing up the transcribed results, as researchers often do, the nature of conversations changed over the life of the project. As trust and understanding grew, so did the depth of sharing and appreciation of the process that was emerging.

The initial ideas of the community grew and developed over the 12-month life of the project. These included the delivery of cooking and dancing ses-sions; however, it also included ideas that would not have been so easy to predict. Gateshead Athletics Stadium is 500 m away from the community hub, but the research revealed that no local people accessed the facility or even knew what was inside. Through contact between the youth worker at Pattinson House and Gateshead Harriers, young people from the estate star-ted accessing groups for the first time. Some have gone on to represent the Harriers in local regional events.

Local people also expressed a desire for their children to walk to school but were concerned about road safety outside the school gates. A local resident led a road traffic campaign, in collaboration with an elected ward councillor, which resulted in changes to the road layout to allow children to walk more safely to school.

Because of the emergent nature of the work, the process was valued as much as the outcomes. It would have been impossible to set out key perfor-mance indicators in advance, as routinely done in public health commission-ing. Given the participatory, iterative nature of the methods, we anticipated the research process would evolve as early findings emerged. This approach presents challenges for conventional academic ethical approval processes and local authority commissioning and performance monitoring 'systems'. It relies on high levels of trust between collaborative partners, and a willingness to take risks, as the possible outcomes, and any unintended consequences, are unclear at the outset.

This was particularly exemplified in the conversations with local school children. Our broad approach to the complex issue of obesity meant that conversations with young people were wide ranging, including discussions of bullying in connection with weight, and community safety concerns, which resulted in young people feeling fearful about accessing local green spaces. This information – although transcribed directly from conversations with young people – was not received favourably by local schools. They had assumed from the focus of the work – childhood obesity – that questioning and conversations would remain very focussed on this one theme. They found it difficult to embrace the emergent nature of the work, and the emphasis on the wider determinants of health, fearing possible criticism about not tackling bullying.

We learned about the importance of clear communication with partners from the outset, and the importance of allowing sufficient time to explore the values and principles underpinning our approach. Our experiences showed the process of emergent change can lead to positive effects in the physical and social environment, as well as attitudinal change among stakeholders, but this is not always an easy process, as Mandy explains:

> It was important not to compromise existing working relationships through the research process, but also to do justice to the research findings by feeding these back to partner organisations in ways that enabled people to act on them. This sometimes felt a tricky balance to achieve.

Through the project, people involved learned to sustain an open-ended exploration and began to notice the way they were generating useful ways of knowing, and acting together as they did so (Wheatley 1992). Through this, we all learned and changed, both individually and collectively. This process makes for fascinating research, as well as profound organisational change.

The presence of the researcher throughout the process was significant, as not only was she able to witness first-hand the activities and capacity building processes that ensued, but also to experience the culture and atmosphere in which the work was undertaken, and to notice the feelings of the individuals involved. As wellbeing is largely about how we feel, a qualitative evaluation that takes account of this emotional context is vital. Some people are critical of this approach as it challenges the traditional 'objectivity' that is often valued so highly within academic circles. However, there is a danger that attempting to maintain 'objectivity' misses an entire dimension of the work that is going on: that of emotional connection. To be effective, ER requires high levels of emotional intelligence among all the collaborating partners, including the ability to have difficult or challenging conversations, change our minds and embrace new ways of thinking.

Much work in disadvantaged communities focusses on encouraging individuals towards independence. However, work with local communities identified people's desire for increased *inter*dependence and connectedness.

> This country's culture ... is based on rugged individualism ... it's what we've been proud of ... and pointed to as our success over the years. And it's fundamentally not working anymore. People like the solutions that come out of a more collective way of operating.
>
> (Phil Cass quoted in Frieze and Wheatley 2011: 31)

This present challenges for research as these concepts are not easily measurable.

By being based in the project on a daily basis, connecting with community, staff and managers in an ongoing way, the researcher was able to actively experience and 'feel' the power of this connectedness and see its effects first-hand through the work of the project, as well as reflecting critically on its effectiveness. Completing the Kolb (1984) learning cycle in this way produces a more rounded approach to learning and understanding (Figure 7.1).

This was not only a process valuable to the researcher:

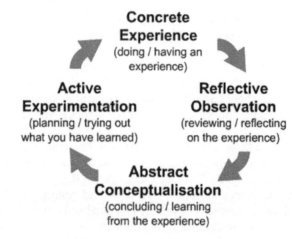

Figure 7.1 Kolb's Learning Cycle.

I found Mandy's presence very helpful, as I had very much been stuck on the 'active experimentation' and 'concrete experience' part of the cycle. I hadn't the time, nor the personal predilection, or the personal discipline or structure to complete the cycle through reflective observation and abstract conceptualisation. Mandy was very experienced in this, and her presence over the year helped me to incorporate these invaluable processes into my own working practice. It therefore helped me to articulate what we were doing so much more clearly, which was really valuable for giving presentations and writing funding bids.

(Sarah Gorman, Edberts House)

An essential ingredient of our partnership was a shared commitment to an asset-based approach; understanding that communities have numerous resources that can contribute to the health and wellbeing of members (Foot and Hopkins 2010). With buy-in and support from senior leadership, the research provided the flexibility to test and learn without pre-defined measures. Focusing on the outcomes that local stakeholders felt were important, identified through 'collective conversations' (Knight et al. 2017) was crucial to the success of the project.

This approach, where ideas or solutions are co-produced, is not always an easy process, as it means that "The future is uncertain and the journey from here to there cannot be known in advance" (Binney et al. 2009: 59); however, the willingness of the partners involved to learn by doing, seem to help. Significant change has emerged as a result; change that has been developed and owned by our community, rather than artificially imposed from 'above' or demanded by a pre-set notion of what the intervention might accomplish.

So much work around childhood obesity that we considered or had read about prior to the launch of the project had taken a structured approach, testing particular interventions or activities. They felt like programmes that were 'done to' the community, removed from the reality of people's daily lives. ER can overcome some of these barriers, by enabling the development of activities which fit the local context. This approach requires the researcher to become 'truly embedded' in the community, becoming involved in community and social events. It takes time and a significant investment of emotional energy. Positive relationships and a huge amount of respect for the community developed over the life of the project, alongside an enhanced understanding of the daily challenges people faced.

Our reflections on what helped

Sharing space / co-location

The embedded researcher spent part of her working week in the community organisation and part with the public health team. A review of the role undertaken by the public health team showed that regular contact with the researcher helped people to "think differently" about how research can be structured to have real-world impact. Improved access to a specialist resource based within the team made a difference:

> I found Mandy's role as an embedded researcher really made me think differently about how I approached my work in terms of the healthy weight agenda. The lived experience of the community made me realise how previous weight management approaches could have been shaped and informed by the community that we were trying to reach. People had no real say or little influence over how services were run and we wondered at the time why we weren't getting the results we needed.
>
> (Emma Gibson, Public Health team)

The benefits of an ER were that the role was seen as providing a neutral and independent "fresh set of eyes". The researcher brought additional research capacity to the public health (PH) team, who saw her as a colleague rather than as an "external consultant". The values, skills and knowledge of the researcher as well as her ability to link staff with other academics across the region, enabled learning to be shared between the PH team and wider colleagues. Providing reflective insights and challenging assumptions, the ER helped inform public health practice, as Mandy found:

> Understanding the context in which people live and work helps to ensure the research is relevant and usable. It increases the likelihood of recommendations being used constructively to make a difference. Asking questions encouraged people to reflect on their work in new ways. Sometimes small changes in attitude can make a big difference in practice.

The right person

The personal qualities of ERs have been identified as key to the success of the role (Marshall et al. 2016; Phipps and Morton 2013). Openness, approachability and excellent communication skills are all words that have been used to describe the researcher by the PH team. Our experience highlights the importance of matching the right person with the right team. The public health team saw the value of qualitative research methods and sought a researcher with these skills. The physical location of the researcher was important. Spending time in the PH office and being welcomed as a part of the team worked well. The researcher was seen as an asset with complementary skills that colleagues could draw on, in different ways, to inform their work. This included being a sounding board, a networker, and a bridge between the Council and wider academic world (Cheetham et al. 2017).

The researcher benefitted from an increased awareness of Council decision-making processes. Understanding the myriad roles of the different groups and committees, proved challenging initially, but also presented an opportunity for learning about potential levers of influence. Feeding in research findings to affect change requires a working understanding of the Council's systems, structures and processes, as well as the personalities of those who work within them. As part of the collaborative process, the PH team provided invaluable help and support in guiding the researcher through this political minefield and navigating bureaucratic reporting and accountability systems.

Understanding the context enabled the researcher to use soft negotiation skills and share learning more effectively with Council colleagues, who were facing a period of organisational uncertainty. This presented challenges and opportunities. There was a willingness to embrace change as staff in the public health team recognised the need for different ways of working, as Emma reflected:

> We are all guilty of spending too much time chained to our desks. Often removed from the realities of the challenges which communities are facing, we are missing the vital link, that community members' experiences need to inform our work. We need to go and out and have conversations. Findings and quotes from both the community and staff show that the Council needs to change its approach. The council is not an expert in someone else's life. We need to listen.

The research findings suggested that the Council could take a broader view and encourage staff to meet people in local communities, extend their knowledge of the area and the challenges facing people, generate and co-produce ideas and support people to create their own solutions in response to local issues.

ER enables the creation and maintenance of positive personal relationships between researchers, policy makers, practitioners and local communities, which have long been recognised as an important way to increase the use of evidence (Lomas 2000). Practical examples of how to do this in public health are limited. The experience of working as a co-located researcher opened opportunities to use formal channels of communication and created informal 'bumping spaces' to tailor messages and maximise impact. It required different kinds of conversational spaces, and only became possible with collaborative partners who were willing to embrace research findings as a catalyst for change. I have had the privilege of learning alongside colleagues open to new and creative ways of thinking in response to deep rooted public health challenges. Change does not happen overnight and a more nuanced understanding of the nature of research impact is needed, as suggested by Rachel Pain and colleagues (2015:4) "Deep co-production is a process often involving a gradual, porous and diffuse series of changes undertaken collaboratively".

Conclusion

Complex public health issues, like childhood obesity, require whole system approaches developed and delivered by multi-agency partnerships, including statutory and voluntary organisations, schools, health services and local communities working together, with evaluation built in. This study contributes to our understanding of ways of engaging communities in efforts to improve health and wellbeing; communities whose voices are not always heard in public health research. The findings contribute to a growing body of research on the role of place in offering opportunities for active engagement, social connection and community participation (Doroud et al. 2018) that are supportive of local communities and involve communities themselves.

Embedded, co-produced research using qualitative, ethnographic and participatory methods revealed new perspectives which would not have been available through quantitative data analysis alone. This approach relies almost entirely on the establishment of trusting, respectful relationships with colleagues and community members.

The findings challenge assumptions that obesity is about individual responsibility. It shows ways in which childhood obesity can be addressed as a collective endeavour. Creating health enhancing environments requires system-wide change, an inclusive, holistic, non-judgemental approach and community focused organisational ethos with robust, visionary leadership. The findings and embedded approach have had real implications for the whole of the council, endorsing asset-based approaches, a focus on the social determinants of health and a need to co-produce solutions in partnership with local communities.

Top tips for successful co-produced research

- Be open, honest, realistic, respectful and responsive
- Jointly negotiate the research questions and methods
- Co-locate researchers in practice settings so they understand the organisational or community context and develop solutions together

- Senior leadership buy-in and support is essential and a willingness to take risks as part of the emergent process of change
- Recognition of the limits of our expertise and a positive dose of bloody mindedness helps too!

References

Blacksher, E. and Lovasi, G. (2012) Place-focused physical activity research, human agency, and social justice in public health: taking agency seriously in studies of the built environment. *Health and Place* Mar;18(2):172–179. doi: doi:10.1016/j.healthplace.2011.08.019. Epub 2011 Sep 10.

Binney, G., Wilke, G. and Williams, C. (2009). *Living leadership.* Harlow, UK: Pearson Education Limited.

Cheetham, M., Wiseman, A., Khazaeli, B., Gibson, E., Gray, P., Van der Graaf, P. and Rushmer, R. (2017) Embedded research: a promising way to create evidence-informed impact in public health? *Journal of Public Health* 40 (suppl.1): i64–i70.

Doroud, N., Fossey, E., and Fortune, T. (2018) Place for being, doing, becoming and belonging: A metasynthesis exploring the role of place in mental health recovery. *Health and Place* 52: 110–120.

Foot, J., & Hopkins, T. (2010) A glass half full: how an asset approach can improve community health and wellbeing. London: Improvement and Development Agency.

Frieze, D. and Wheatley, M. (2011, Fall). It's time for the heroes to go home. *Leader to Leader*: 27–32.

Gateshead Council Joint Strategic Needs Assessment (2018) *Obesity and excess weight.* https://www.gatesheadjsna.org.uk/article/6211/Headline-data accessed 23. 11. 18

Government Office for Science (2007) *Foresight. Tackling obesities: Future choices summary of key messages* https://www.gov.uk/government/collections/tackling-obesities-future-choices

Holmes, B., Best, A., Davies, H., Hunter, D., Kelly, M.P., Marshall, M., and Rycroft-Malone, J. (2017) Mobilising knowledge in complex health systems: a call to action. *Evidence and Policy Evidence & Policy* 13(3): 539–560s https://doi.org/10.1332/174426416X14712553750311

Knight, A.D., Lowe, T., Brossard, M. and Wilson, J. (2017) *A whole new world: funding and commissioning in complexity.* Newcastle-upon-Tyne and London: Newcastle University and Collaborate.

Kolb, D. (1984). *Experiential learning: experience as the source of learning and development. Englewood Cliffs.* New Jersey: Prentice Hall.

Lomas, J. (2000) Using linkage and exchange to move research into policy at a Canadian foundation. *Health Aff.* 19(3):236–240.

Marmot, M. (2010) *Marmot Review final report: strategic review of health inequalities in England post 2010.* London: Department of Health.

Marshall, M., Eyre, L., Lalani, M., Khan, S., Mann, S., de Silva, D., and Shapiro, J. (2016) Increasing the impact of health service research on service improvement: the researcher-in-residence model. *Royal Society of Medicine* 109(6): 220–225.

McGinity, R., & Salokangas, M. (2014) Introduction: 'embedded research' as an approach into academia for emerging researchers *Management in Education* 28(1): 3–5.

Pain, R., Askins, K., Banks, S., Cook, T., Crawford, G., Crookes, L., Darby, S., Heslop, J., Holden, A., Houston, M., Jeffes, J., Lambert, Z., McGlen, L., McGlynn, C., Ozga, J., Raynor, R., Robinson, Y., Shaw, S., Stewart, C., and Vanderhoven, D. (2015) *Mapping alternative impact. Alternative approaches to impact from co-pro-duced research*, Durham University Centre for Social Justice and Community Action   https://www.dur.ac.uk/socialjustice/researchprojects/mapping-alt-impact/ accessed 21. 11. 18

Phipps, D. and Morton, S. (2013) Qualities of knowledge brokers: reflections from practice *Evidence and Policy* 3(9):255–265

Rycroft-Malone, J. (2014) From knowing to doing – from the academy to practice *International Journal of Health Policy Making* 2(1): 45–46.

South, J. (2017) *A guide to community-centred approaches for health and wellbeing. Full report*. London: Public Health England. https://assets.publishing.service.gov.uk/gov ernment/uploads/system/uploads/attachment_data/file/417515/A_guide_to_communi ty-centred_approaches_for_health_and_wellbeing__full_report_.pdf

Vindrola-Padros, C., Pape, T., Utley, M. and Fulop, N. (2017) The role of embedded research in quality improvement: a narrative review. *BMJ Qual Saf* 26: 70–80

Wheatley, M. (1992) *Leadership and the new science: Learning about organization from an orderly universe*. San Francisco, CA: Berrett-Koehler Publishers, Inc.

Whitehead, M., Pennington, A., Orton, L., Nayak, S., Petticrew, M., Sowden, A., and White, M. (2016) How could differences in 'control over destiny' lead to socio-eco-nomic inequalities in health? A synthesis of theories and pathways in the living environment. *Health and Place* 39: 51–61.

8 Co-producing a story of recovery

A Books Beyond Words book group

Jane Bourne

Introduction

There are approximately 1.5 million people in the UK who have an intellectual disability (Mental Health Foundation 2018), which is defined by the Department of Health (Department of Health 2009) as a "significant reduced ability to understand new or complex information, to learn new skills (impaired intelligence), with a reduced ability to cope independently (impaired social functioning), which started before adulthood" (p. 14). These individuals are amongst the most socially excluded and mistreated groups in Great Britain, and often need on-going daily support from family, carers and/ or support teams. At any one time 40% of adults with an intellectual disability diagnosis also has a mental health difficulty (England.nhs.uk 2017). In 2017, NHS England's Transforming Care Agenda aimed to change this as they ensured better mental health care in the community and making sure any admissions to hospital were as short as possible. Unfortunately, recent figures from MENCAP (Mencap 2018) still show an inadequacy in community services in terms of both quality and access particularly around integration into communities. This has meant that many people continue to be at risk of the revolving door back to hospital (Gamie 2018).

Hospital admissions unfortunately do happen, and once people are ready for discharge this can be another challenge (England.nhs.uk 2017). Hospital settings can offer some people reassurance and make them feel safe; as they become comfortable seeing the same people and know the regular ward rounds and routine of activities. When it is time to return to the community, where a person first became unwell, it can provoke some anxiety. Having a well-planned discharge pathway can alleviate some of these worries attached to discharges and offer a person some confidence and reassurance that they will be supported (Head et al. 2018). By gently exposing people to a community facility, where they are able to meet similar people, as part of their weekly routine, normalises a community environment and can prepare people for discharge (Ager et al. 2001). Therefore, the forming of community partnerships between staff from an in-patient Treatment and Assessment Unit, past patients and a local library was helpful in supporting people returning to

living in the community. The benefits of past patients being part of the production meant that as they had themselves followed this pathway they could
support current patients through a peer support role, due to their own lived
experiences.

Partnerships for developing 'bridging'

'The Book Group', as an initiative, was first developed by Northumberland,
Tyne and Wear NHS Foundation Trust (NTW) in partnership with Hebburn
Community Library, which is located within walking distance of an adult
inpatient Assessment and Treatment unit. Developing partnerships between
different working sectors, such as the public and cultural sectors, and the
voluntary and independent sectors, has been of great benefit in supporting
'community bridging' (Hackett & Bourne 2014). Low-cost accessible community space is often problematic for the NHS to fund outside hospitals and
since the theme to community bridging is linking to the community, the
development of relationships and partnerships outside the NHS and NHS
property is a priority (Sutton & Gates 2018). Co-producing a model of care
between in-patient services and a partnership with an accessible community
facility such as the library meant that people could be safely supported, and
'bridged', directly into the heart of a community (Hackett & Bourne 2014).

The library is in South Tyneside, near Newcastle; it is a new build, with a
café, swimming pool and leisure suit; and seen as hub for the local community. The library is part of the 'Safe Place' scheme, which is aimed at helping
adults with all kinds of disabilities handle day-to-day challenges like reading
and writing, being bullied and needing help or even something as simple as
forgetting where they left their mobile phone or wallet. The intention of the
scheme is to make it easy for vulnerable adults to find 'safe places' they can
easily access, which can offer long-term supportive networks (Keyes & Brandon 2012). As a venue the library was ideal for this community-bridging
project.

The library when approached with idea of 'The Book Group' was enthusiastic
and eager to support the project. They initially purchased 15 copies of ten independent titles, from the Books Beyond Words series that were seen as the most
suitable (see Table 8.1). They offered a private room, with tea and coffee facilities
on a weekly basis for ten weeks, without cost. Visiting the library allowed the group
to familiarise themselves with library staff over the ten weeks, who assisted people
in feeling comfortable, so they felt able to access the library when the group was not
running. The idea of the facility being a 'safe place' with familiar people also
allowed people to reach out and build positive relationships. This partnership
development meant that the libraries membership also grew, and their ongoing
inclusiveness agenda was met.

Apart from people accessing the book group, the library invited everyone
who attended to enter a Six Book Challenge. This is a scheme run by The
Reading Agency (Reading Agency 2019), which takes place each year in

Table 8.1 Book titles

1	*Making friends*
2	*Food, fun, healthy and safe*
3	*Mugged*
4	*A new home in the community*
5	*The drama group*
6	*Speaking up for myself*
7	*Feeling cross and sorting it out*
8	*Exercise*
9	*Falling in love*
10	*George gets smart*

libraries, colleges, workplaces and prisons. The challenge invited group members to read six books, review them and enter prize drawers, which all of them did, in the form of the Books Beyond Words series with pictures, audio books or, when people were able to, reading books (Hollins 2016). The library offered people some autonomy and a place visit independently and access different accessible books, music and films, which many had never done before. Each book group member, including facilitators and support staff:

- Became a library member
- Took part in the 'six book challenge'
- Used a range of library resources in addition to the book group books, such as audio books and picture books.
- Accessed the internet

'The books'

The resources for the group from the Books Beyond Words series, were developed for people with an intellectual disability, by people with intellectual disabilities on topics relevant to their needs. They were first produced by Psychiatrist Baroness Sheila Hollins, as an aide for individuals who find reading difficult, but can understand pictures. Information about the books can be found on their website. Each book tells a story through the pictures, linked to the title. The book group's facilitators were a registered dramatherapist, who had some independent training from the Books Beyond Words trainers on how to use the books, and a Positive Behaviour Support Nurse. Both facilitators were based at the hospital and both were familiar with group members, from the hospital and the community. The book group ran weekly, and people supported each other to share a story together through the use of pictures. Each group member was invited to speak about a page in the book autonomously, so as to help with confidence building, turn-taking skills, concentration, participation and communication. The ten titles that were read throughout the course of the ten-week pilot program can be seen in Table 8.1. The titles often started a dialogue about the subject between the group.

Aim of the research

The project was co-produced to offer a gradual exposure to the community for people with an intellectual disability and mental health difficulty who were ready for discharge from a Treatment and Assessment Unit. The research had three aims:

- To see if friendships between people in hospital and people living in the community, who had similar transitional lived experiences, could help support a peer's discharge.
- To understand if the shared narratives that allowed people to reflect on personal experiences through the context of the different stories were helpful in bringing people together.
- To identify if the strength of a community setting such as a library could offer an immediate and long-term supportive environment for vulnerable adults.

Methods for evaluation

The main source of data collection was through interviews, which were with: current and past patients, who were supported by staff if needed, support staff who attended the group and the library staff. Using qualitative research gives the maximum opportunity to learn from peoples' perceptions and experiences (Richie & Lewis 2003). It seeks to answer the questions such as 'What is going on here?' and to get descriptions in detail of what is happening in a specific community and it can offer a lived experience around a phenomenon (Paley 2018). The focus of this research was to explore if we could co-produce this kind of group and what participating in the group offered people.

An evaluation of the books as individual stories was also completed alongside the research. This was done at the end of each group session, when each book was rated using a rating scale from one to ten. The number scale was placed on the floor as a visual aid to help people with this process (Table 8.2). Group members were invited to either stand on the number they rated the book or call out the number from their seat. Comments linking with these scores, in relation to both the book and the development of the group story, were also discussed and documented.

Table 8.2 Group average book ratings

Books	Ratings
1. *Making friends*	6
2. *Food, fun, healthy and safe*	6.2
3. *Mugged*	8.7
4. *A new home in the community*	4.9
5. *Drama group*	9
6. *Speaking up for myself*	5.1
7. *Feeling cross and sorting it out*	6.3
8. *Exercise*	9
9. *Falling in love*	7.7

Twenty people were interviewed for the research project and invitations were extended to everyone who had attended the group. Each interview lasted half an hour and each interview was recorded and transcribed with confidential identifiers coded to anonymise the group members. Interviews followed a semi-structured topic guide with open-ended questions. It is understood that open-ended questions can enable people with an intellectual disability to participate in research much more easily; although this is subject to an individuals' communication skills (Porter & Lacey 2005). Also, using open-ended questions can produce more accurate data from people with an intellectual disability as it can change the tendency to recall words most recently used by the interviewer (Kroese et al. 1998). Additional data was also obtained from field notes gathered from the NHS facilitators. Consent for the research was obtained from everyone involved.

Data analysis

The collected data was analysed using framework analysis. This is an interpretive process where data is systematically searched (Richie & Lewis 2003). Analytical frameworks such as this approach can emphasise the transparency of the analysis process (Braun & Clarke 2013). A series of interconnected stages enable the researcher to move back and forth across the data until a coherent interpretation of themes emerge (Smith & Firth 2011). NVivo qualitative research software (Bazeley 2013) was also used. This is fully compatible with a framework analysis approach and was employed to support the data management and analysis process. Some of themes were initially identified from the research aim and field notes and then refined throughout the analysis process to reflect the emerging data.

Results

The findings are organized using themes: (a) Working together, (b) On-going support, (c) Increased social networks, (d) Story sharing.

Working together

The first theme was 'working together'. People with an intellectual disability do not always feel valued but being involved in research projects has been seen to help people's self-worth (Inglis & Cook 2011). Working together, being part of a group and developing the project helped people feel they were contributing to something and supporting other people through their own experiences (Milner & Kelly 2009). One person spoke about this and described how their own confidence had built due to supporting other people from the group:

> People think that because I sometimes need support I cannot support other people, but I can.

Another person reflected on how important the group had helped her but also how she had seen improvements in others:

> This group has helped me with my confidence, and I can see that it has helped other people too … they seem more confident now.

Working together to form the group, having fun, meeting new people and experiencing something new where all discussed as being positive aspects of the project:

> I didn't realise that reading a picture book together would make me laugh so much.
> I could see the topic 'making friends' is important to everyone here including me.

On-going support

The second theme, 'on-going support', was vast in its meaning. It included sub themes: travel, getting to the group, feeling anxious, new skills and somewhere to go. These different kinds of 'on-going support' were recognised by the group and discussed individually, dependent on different people's experiences, stages of recovery, physical health and geographic distance from the library. For example, one person felt she was much better and more confident living in the community, but still needed some practical help to get to the group. Transport was found at times to be challenging and often a barrier to people attending the group; physical disabilities, costs and/or lack of support where all discussed. Accessing groups in general, once living in the community, was discussed as being 'a problem' at times due to commuting difficulties:

> I probably wouldn't have been able to come today if I hadn't been picked up.
>   The other week I got a lift but this week I found it hard to come and I needed to travel by two buses.

Linking with other group members became a positive strategy so that people could share transport to come to the group. The process, although challenging to arrange in itself, due to planning, was also seen as a supportive measure as it helped to further develop friendships.

> Travelling together means we have become friends and talk more.

This theme of 'ongoing support' also included receiving regular reassurance and getting feedback from people, as one group member shared:

> I think that knowing I was supported and hearing I was doing OK made me not give up ... it's not always easy.

A mutual support model that offers a laying of support (Keyes & Brandon 2012) helps people feel better due to an understanding of commonality of people's experiences and circumstances. One patient from the hospital expressed this model in a simplified way.

> I like seeing my friend here it makes me look forward to coming ... she is supportive, and she knows what it is like for me.

Increased social networks

The group environment meant that friendships and relationships were developed over the ten weeks between everyone involved in the project. This was a topic of conversation discussed in the interviews, which developed into the theme 'increased social networks'. The project had enabled a place for people to go and visit, a place that offered a safe environment where people felt welcome and valued.

> I feel that I know people at the library ... I can just turn up and feel welcome.

People who had previously had an admission but were now settled in the community visited the group to link in with professionals, friendships they had made whilst in hospital and to help support people on their own discharge pathway. This offered them a wider network and made them feel valued.

> I think going to the group shows I am helping people in the hospital and they know it is possible to leave.

The library environment meant that people over time developed relationships with other people who worked at the library and café and also people who visited but were not part of the project.

> I seem to know everyone now … everyone says hello to me … it makes me feel good.

Story sharing

The theme 'story sharing' had a few connotations. Sharing stories at the group using the Books Beyond Words series was seen as a way to collectively share a story that the group produced together through deciding what the pictures meant. This was a really positive experience and helped people to open up not only about themselves but also gave them some confidence to speak up in front of the group and offer a suggestion of what a picture within the story might mean. One person spoke about this experience.

> When I first went to the group I just sat there thinking that if I said anything people might laugh at me … slowly I felt better and then I made lots of suggestions … all the time.

Box 8.1 Feedback from 'The Drama Book' read at the book group

Sharing and building a story was discussed as being fun, confidence building, skills building such as turn-taking and reflective. Box 8.1 shows some of the feedback from one of the books after a story was developed together at the group.

K – I liked the way people got introduced to each other – 8

C – Interesting book really liked all of it – 9

S – The hero was good. Thought the drama group could have given him more confidence – 5

G – Really enjoyed the book – I like the main character – 9

J – I thought at times it was funny – 10

T – I liked it because the main character started going to a see a show and then tried it out for himself – 10

A – I really loved the happy ending – 9

AT – Main character was great he was the main character in the book and then in the play –10

S – Good sharing and confidence building book – 9

SB – Liked how the main character went from been nervous to then playing the lead -10

SS – The book made everyone think about the group – 10

J – I really enjoyed this book my favorite so far – I liked the way that the character slowly built his confidence – 9

The story telling theme also related to sharing people's own experiences. The books and the stories often communicated real-life experiences, desires and difficulties. People at the group through telling stories processed events and started sharing personal information. Support workers learnt difficulties a person was experiencing but had been unable to share to anyone.

> The story about 'making friends' was really important and I learnt that she wanted to make more friends now she is feeling much better … I am trying to find places we can go and do that.

Discussion

The importance of the on-going support and collaboration with everyone involved in a person's care, including the person with a learning disability is emphasized as crucial for morale and confidence (Mascha 2007). The reduction in hospital beds and changes made due to the Transforming Care Agenda has meant that people need to be better supported in the community (England.nhs.uk 2017) with an emphasis on prevention and early intervention to avoid re-occurring hospital admissions. Having a place that offers on-going support and somewhere to go that is familiar, free and supportive for people once living in the community is an important intervention for keeping well and to help stop the rotating door back into hospital.

Group activities can assist in building confidence, self-esteem and positive relationships in people with learning disabilities (Beail 2016). On a hospital ward groups are accessed daily and seen as part of the treatment program. However, once people are discharged, similar groups are not always accessible, due to reasons such as cost, travel, lack of motivation, enthusiasm or people not wanting to engage or feeling anxious at meeting new people. Friendships, positive relationships and feeling part of something are normal human desires but are often more difficult for people with intellectual disabilities to achieve. This can mean that they become at risk of loneliness, isolation, low mood and the lack of behavioural rewards. 'The Book Group' as a project helped to re-engage people into the community through a slow exposure to the environment. The familiar group environment transported into the community, facilitated by familiar people and mutually supported by staff and peers made the experience this experience less anxiety provoking.

People with learning disabilities and mental health and/or behaviours that challenge are often socially isolated having fewer friends and fewer opportunities for socialising than the general population (Department of Health 2001). We know that having time together with similar people who have had similar lived experiences is a way to develop friendships and build trusting relationships (Kroese et al. 2012). For people ready for discharge moving into the community can be inherently difficult, frightening and lonely. So, building a supportive graded network in the local community can help support relationship building and the forming of alliances which in turn can help build people's confidence (Salmon et al. 2013). Sustaining friendships is 'consistently shown as being one of the greatest challenges faced by learning disability services' (Department of Health 2001). Although there are barriers relating to transport and travel, the project offered people a time and space to meet and share an experience and be part of a developing social network.

Having support staff as part of the group was a positive aspect of the project. Staff have often spoke about constraints in the environment such as tight schedules, meal planning and staff changes (Salmon et al. 2013), which has meant that accessing external resources where people with learning disabilities can meet similar people to themselves and widen their network is difficult to facilitate. Opportunities for this to happen, where time is put aside to actively be involved together in an activity can usually be difficult to achieve (Kroese et al. 2012). Even though we know that staff spending time with those they support; taking a direct interest in them rather than doing task related jobs, can avoid mental health crises from occurring (Salmon et al. 2013). Therefore, due to the co-production of the project, it meant that everyone was involved in working together to achieve the book group's success and this meant being active and present in the activity so that relationships between everyone could be developed.

Conclusion

Mental health services for adults with learning disabilities and mental health difficulties and/or behaviour that challenges have improved in recent years with many new guidelines and policies setting out ways of working. But flexibility and opportunities for people to be supported in different ways in the heart of communities are fundamental if the transforming care agenda is to be successful. The book group as a bridging project to help people move from hospital to the community was successful in helping people to feel they had a network they could access, receive on-going support from and a group that made them to feel valued. Transport can be a barrier to attending groups, but when links are made that facilitate commuting with peers this can further develop relationships and friendships. Quotes from members of the group illustrate the benefit of this kind of co-production community model and its potential emancipatory affects through mutual and peer support.

Learning

The weekly group helped people slowly integrate back into the community and gave past patients a chance to attend when they felt isolated or at risk of being unwell, so that they could share their feelings and communicate with their peers, who have similar lived experiences. This allowed a network of mutual and peer support to develop.

Recommendations/future planning

Further evaluation

We would like to see if attending the book group improves people's self-esteem and will ask people to complete an adapted version of the 'Rosenberg Self-Esteem Scale' before and after completing ten weeks of book club. Further development of the book group could eventually lead to a separate group for members who wish to try their hand at storytelling and story making themselves, giving them the opportunity to tell their own stories to others in a new way.

Five tips

Five tips for developing this kind of project are:

- Encourage peer support as it is powerful in recovery. When people with a lived experience share their stories, it can inspire others to see alternative possibilities.
- Link and build partnerships with local community agencies as it can mean obtaining room space outside a hospital setting is less problematic.
- Finding a central accessible location, and slowly introducing people to attend, can develop safe relationships with the staff who work there; this, in turn, can enable a place for people to visit whenever they feel isolated and/or vulnerable.
- Use a mutual support model, a form of layering, as this can allow everyone to feel supported.
- Urge all who attend the group to be active members, no matter what role they have, as this can be helpful in developing positive relationships between staff and the people they support.

Four more community book groups are now running independently, after the library asked if the facilitator could offer training to facilitators in the private sector. Training is on-going so that more book groups can be developed within the area for people with learning disabilities.

- Four additional book groups are now running independently, locally as a result of the partnership work, although not linked to the hospital.
- Training and guidance has been given to new group facilitators from NHS staff on using the books.
- Books have been taken from the library to the in-patient unit independently when patients have been too unwell to visit the library.
- A nomination for an 'Excellence Award'.
- Ten more titles purchased.
- The room space has been extended to be used on weekly basis as needed.

This project shows the benefits of building community partnerships to help transitions from hospital to living back in the community, insofar as establishing a feeling of belonging. It looks at the use of The Books Beyond Words series for a bridging group, the development of the group and of similar groups and the implications for future practice.

References

Ager, A., Myers, F., Kerr, P., Myles, S. and Green, A. (2001). Moving home: Social integration for adults with intellectual disabilities resettling into community provision. *Journal of Applied Research in Intellectual Disabilities*, 14(4), 392–400.

Bazeley, P. (2013. *Qualitative data analysis*. London: Sage.

Beail, N. (Ed.). (2016). *Psychological therapies and people who have intellectual disabilities*. Retrieved from British Psychological Society website:/system/files/Public%20files/id_ therapies.pdf

Books Beyond Words (2019). *Beyond words empowering people through picture*. https://booksbeyondwords.co.uk/bookshop/ [Accessed 9 Feb. 2019].

Braun, V., & Clarke, V. (2013). *Successful qualitative research*. Los Angeles: SAGE

Department of Health (2009). *Valuing people now: A new three-year strategy for people with learning disabilities*. London: Crown.

Department of Health. (2001). *Valuing people – a new strategy for learning disability for the 21st century*. [online] Available at: https://www.gov.uk/government/publications/valuing-people-a-new-strategy-for-learning-disability-for-the-21st-century [Accessed 22 Apr. 2018].

England.nhs.uk. (2015). *Transforming care for people with learning disabilities – next steps*. [online] Available at: https://www.england.nhs.uk/wp-content/uploads/2015/01/transform-care-nxt-stps.pdf [Accessed 22 Apr. 2018].

England.nhs.uk. (2017). *Transforming care agenda*. [online] Available at: https://www.england.nhs.uk/wp-content/uploads/2017/02/model-service-spec-2017.pdf [Accessed 7 Apr. 2018].

Gamie, J. (2018). *Flagship learning difficulty programme branded a "failure"*. Retrieved from https://www.hsj.co.uk/quality-and-performance/flagship-learning-difficulty-programme-branded-a-failure/7022834.article

Hackett, S., & Bourne, J. (2014). The get going group: Dramatherapy with adults who have learning disabilities and mental health difficulties. *Dramatherapy*, 36(1), 43–50. https://doi.org/10.1080/02630672.2014.909981.

Head, A., Ellis-Caird, H., Rhodes, L., & Parkinson, K. (2018). Transforming identities through Transforming Care: How people with learning disabilities experience moving out of hospital. *British Journal Of Learning Disabilities, 46*(1), 64–70. doi: doi:10.1111/bld.12213.

Hollins, S. (2016). Looking beyond learning disabilities. *BMJ*, i3572. doi: doi:10.1136/bmj.i3572.

Inglis, P., & Cook, T. (2011). Ten top tips for effectively involving people with a learning disability in research. *Journal Of Learning Disabilities And Offending Behaviour, 2*(2), 98–104. doi: doi:10.1108/20420921111152441

Keyes, S. E., and T. Brandon. (2012. Mutual support: A model of participatory support by and for people with learning difficulties. *British Journal of Learning Disabilities* 40(3): 222–228. doi:10.1111/j.1468-3156.2011.00698.x

Kroese, B., Gillott, A., and Atkinson, V. (1998) Consumers with intellectual disabilities as service evaluators. *Journal of Applied Research in Intellectual Disabilities*, 11(2), 116–128.

Kroese, B., Rose, J., Heer, K. and O'Brien, A. (2012). Mental health services for adults with intellectual disabilities – what do service users and staff think of them?. *Journal of Applied Research in Intellectual Disabilities*, 26(1), 3–13.

Mascha, K. (2007). Staff morale in day care centres for adults with intellectual disabilities. *Journal of Applied Research in Intellectual Disabilities*, 20(3), 191–199.

Mencap. (2018). *What is a learning disability?*. [online] Available at: https://www.mencap.org.uk/learning-disability-explained/what-learning-disability [Accessed 10 Apr. 2018].

Mental Health Foundation. (2018). *Learning disability statistics | Mental Health Foundation*. [online] Available at: https://www.mentalhealth.org.uk/learning-disabilities/help-information/learning-disability-statistics- [Accessed 23 Apr. 2018].

Milner, P. and Kelly, B. (2009). Community participation and inclusion: People with disabilities defining their place. *Disability & Society*, 24(1), 47–62.

Paley, J. (2018). Meaning, lived experience, empathy and boredom: Max van Manen on phenomenology and Heidegger. *Nursing Philosophy*, 19(3), e12211. doi: doi:10.1111/nup.12211

Porter, J. and Lacey, P. (2005) *Researching learning difficulties: A guide for practitioners*. London: Paul Chapman Publishing.

Reading Agency. (2019). The Reading Agency Website. Retrieved from https://readingagency.org.uk/adults

Richie, J., & Lewis, J. (Eds.) (2003). *Qualitative research practice: A guide for social science students & researchers*. London: Sage.

Salmon, R., Holmes, N. and Dodd, K. (2013. Reflections on change: supporting people with learning disabilities in residential services. *British Journal of Learning Disabilities*, 42(2), 141–152.

Smith, J., & Firth, J. (2011) Qualitative data analysis: Application of the framework approach. *Nurse Researcher*, 18(2), 52–62.

Sutton, P., & Gates, B. (2018) Giving voice to adults with intellectual disabilities and experience of mental ill-health: Validity of psychosocial approach. *Nurse Researchers*. Sept 26(2), 19–26.

9 How do we co-produce research in the prison environment?

Jennifer Ferguson, Aisha Holloway, Victoria Guthrie and Dorothy Newbury-Birch

Introduction

This chapter considers undertaking research in a prison environment. Co-production has proved essential when working with prison staff and prisoners, and the PRISM-A project (mentioned in detail below) highlighted this. This chapter will talk through some facts around the prison environment, some experience from the PRISM-A project, and end with some useful tips for those wishing to undertake research in a similar environment.

Prison environment

Globally, there are over 10 million people incarcerated, with prisoners bearing a substantial burden of communicable and non-communicable diseases (Fazel and Baillargeon 2011). Since the 1940s there has been an increasing trend in the number of individuals incarcerated in the UK. In August 2018, there were 86,000 people in prison and young offender institutions. The cost of prisons to the Ministry of Justice (MoJ) was £3.954 billion in 2016–2017.

Due to changes in organisation, Her Majesty's Prison and Probation Service (HMPPS) replaced the National Offender Management Service (NOMS) on 1 April 2017 (Office 2017). Since this time, NOMS has ceased to exist and its functions were split between HMPPS and the MoJ. HMPPS retained responsibility for the operational management of prisons, while responsibility for the commissioning and policy has moved to the ministry. HMPPS is an executive agency and is responsible for the prison estate, including adult prisons (both male and female), youth offender institutions and some immigration removal services.

Prison population

The fact that men are responsible for the majority of offending behaviour, is undisputed. The arrest data is released annually by the MoJ to prove this point. There are 131 male prisons in the UK, and 13 extra contracted prisons (Mah et al. 2018). The prison population is a constantly growing population.

The prison population in general in England and Wales has quadrupled in size between 1900 and 2017; and in Scotland the prison population has almost doubled. Northern Ireland prisons have seen an increase in the prison population since 2000, by 38%; although their prison population is currently at its lowest since 2010 (Library 2018). To place some context to those figures, in England and Wales for every 100,000 of the population, 179 are prisoners (both male and female); Scotland, 166, and Northern Ireland, 98. In terms of male prisoners, in England and Wales there are 348 male prisoners for every 100,000 men in the entire population (in 2016/2017). This is a substantial increase from 1900, where there were 152 for every 100,000 men (Ministry of Justice 2018).

Risky behaviours

As with most organisational transformations, cost have been reduced and the funding from the Ministry to NOMS, now HMPPS, reduced by 13% (from 2009–2010 to 2016–2017) and whilst the prison population has remained broadly stable (between 83,852 and 87,080), NOMS reduced the number of operational staff in public prisons by 30% to manage within the reduced budget. The National Audit Office Report (Office 2017) highlighted that the issues the Ministry are looking out for due to all of the change are: the Prison Estate Transformation Programme due to the number of prisons that have been deemed not fit for purpose; staff recruitment and retention; prison safety and security, which has declined since 2012; and finally the mental health of prisoners due to the number of suicides in the estate.

Safety in prisons is declining and the number of assaults has increased from 29,485 by 13% in one year (NPC 2012). The number of serious assaults has increased by 10% (2,856) and the assaults on members of staff by 23% (8,429). Interestingly, however, the number of suicides has fallen from 115, to 69; however, that is still a high amount of suicides. The prevalence of risky drinking in the prison system is between 59% and 63% whilst the levels of probable dependency are between 36% and 43% (Newbury-Birch et al. 2018). Similarly, there is a high prevalence of drug use. Research in the criminal justice system (in prison in particular) around alcohol is sparse (Sondhi et al. 2016; Newbury-Birch et al. 2018), but a growing area of interest, and a number of studies have started to look at alcohol use disorders and screening and brief interventions in the criminal justice system (Newbury-Birch et al. 2009; Coulton et al. 2012; Newbury-Birch et al. 2014; Newbury-Birch et al. 2016a).

Health and social care

The health of prisoners is now considered a public health issue. This is a new change due to the Health and Social Care Act 2012. Section 15(1)(c) requires the Board to commission certain health services "for persons who are detained in a prison or in other accommodation of a prescribed description".

This caused the public health system to change; in order to deliver the Government's commitment to "improve the health of the poorest, fastest" (Government. 2012).

Alcohol brief interventions for male remand prisoners: protocol for a complex intervention framework development and feasibility study (PRISM-A)

The PRISM-A study (Holloway et al. 2017), an MRC funded project, took place in 2016 across two prisons, one in the North East of England, and one in Scotland. The aim was to explore the feasibility and acceptability of an ABI for adult remand, male prisoners; to develop an appropriate ABI for such prisoners; and to prepare a protocol for a multi-centre randomised pilot study. The project was aligned to the early phase of the Medical Research Councils (MRC) framework for the development and evaluation of complex interventions (Craig et al. 2008). The study comprised three stages, using mixed methods, and separate recruitment for prison stakeholders in stage 2.

Stage 1

The aim of stage 1 was to identify the prevalence of self-reported hazardous/harmful alcohol consumption in adult male prisoners. Prevalence was measured using the gold standard Alcohol Use Disorder Identification Test (AUDIT) (Babor et al. 1989) screening tool. This allows an individual to be categorised as either a harmful, hazardous or dependent drinker by completing 10 screening questions and giving a simple score. The possibility of a potential alcohol use disorder is determined by a score from 0–40 and the categories are split from 0–7, 8–15, 16–19 and 20+. A score of 8 or more suggests is considered a potential alcohol use disorder. The AUDIT and reported views of ABIS delivered in prisons with acceptability of participation in a future ABI study with follow up. Research Assistants (RAs) carried out this element of the study using a questionnaire. The study aimed to recruit 250 adult male remand prisoners in each prison site, aged 18 or over, incarcerated for less than three months, and willing to provide informed consent. Written consent was obtained by the RAs and the questionnaire included the AUDIT, and questions experiences or opinions of receiving alcohol advice or information, their willingness to receive it and whether or not they would be willing to take part in a study involving a follow up element. Questions were read out and answers recorded by the RA on a hard copy.

Stage 2

The aim of stage 2 was to complete some qualitative interviews to first understand the feasibility and acceptability amongst adult remand prisoners of an ABI designed for them. Second, the qualitative work aimed to explore their perspectives in relation to their: beliefs and perceptions about their alcohol use, views regarding the acceptability of receiving an ABI whilst on remand, experiences of engaging with health professionals in relation to their alcohol use, the nature of this and the perceived impact and outcome of it, and finally their perceptions of acceptable alcohol screening, intervention delivery points and techniques, methods of delivery, and by whom.

Twenty male remand prisoners across two study sites were interviewed. Each participant was shown an infographic outlining the key components and the nature of an ABI. A focus group was also held at each site to explore prison stakeholders perceptions of the feasibility and acceptability of an ABI with this population. Focus groups were facilitated again by the RAs and were structured by a topic guide, informed by the qualitative data collected in stage 2.

Stage 3

Stage 3 involved identifying what an adapted intervention mapped self-efficacy enhancing ABI looks like. This was done using data collected and analysed in stages 1 and 2. Intervention mapping was used to refine and develop an existing self-efficacy enhancing ABI (Kok et al. 2016) to reduce reported levels of alcohol consumption in male remand prisoners. This was undertaken by members of the research study group, with activity and input form the Expert Advisory Group.

The results of the PRISM-A project showed that this type of research can be carried out in prisons. However, through the qualitative work, especially with staff and stakeholders, it became apparent that working alongside the staff in prison was essential. More time than was anticipated had to be put into working out the different regimes in each prison, and learning which members of staff needed to be involved in different ways. For example, it could not have been anticipated how vital it would be to work with peer prisoners. Putting the time into working *with* the relevant staff, as opposed to alongside them, made a significant difference in how the project worked.

Differing prisons in PRISM-A

It is important to note that although all prison establishments are very similar in terms of the environment; regimes differ depending upon what the Governor has established in any given prison. This became very apparent in the PRISM-A study. Some examples of this are included below.

One RA had keys, the other did not, which meant having to be escorted by already busy prison officers. Given the prison environment, and the amount of locked gates and doors, this can hold up research activity significantly. Not to mention, going to the bathroom. Another difference was that one RA could only data collect in the mornings only, the other all day. The RA with keys could only have access to prisoners before 12pm. However, that researcher had keys and could potentially survey 15–20 prisoners in this time. The other could have access to prisoners all day, but given the complication of being escorted, could survey the same amount, in double the time. Peer prisoners, often called "Listeners" or "PIDS workers" introduced the study for one RA, and proved very helpful. The peer prisoners had more time to work closely with the RA and the prisoners interacted with them very well, therefore taking an interest in the study. At the other site, peer prisoners were not used as part of the research study, therefore more work had to be done with staff to ensure everyone understood the study and purpose of the RA being there. At the second site, a lot of every day was taken up explaining this again to the new staff on duty.

Another difference between sites was that, at one, all data collection took place on one wing, the first night centre. At the second site, data was collected from various different places on the prison estate. This, unfortunately, was the site that the RA did not have keys, therefore the amount of time spent data collecting amounted to a lot more at the second site. The final difference was that one prison was mostly remand, meaning there was a high turnover of prisoners, which subsequently is brilliant for data collecting with new prisoners. The other site held both remand and sentenced prisoners, meaning more time was spent determining eligibility for the study, as only those who had incarcerated for less than three months could take part in the study.

As described, it is apparent that having keys, having peer prisoners assisting with the project, and being a remand only setting made the data collection more straight forward for one of the RAs. Both prison sites had an extremely strong co-production approach, which was called upon a number of times in the second site. When difficulties arose due to the RA's lack of keys, the Governor was called to assist with any difficulties, and they were soon ironed out.

However, the data collecting element is merely one part of conducting a research study in a prison. As mentioned in more detail below, setting up the project, and the various training also differs across different prison sites, and the RA who had more straightforward circumstances data collecting, had more rigorous training to undertake than the second RA, partly because of having access to keys, but also, simply the difference in demands from the two prisons.

Training and preparation

As would be expected, a researcher will come against a number of barriers when wanting to conduct research in a prison. There are obviously rigorous ethical applications to consider, and the issue of security. There are also a number of various training exercises to complete before being able to work in the environment, even as a researcher, even for a short period of time. The training exercises are exactly the same as those that other staff have to complete, and are undertaken alongside new members of staff which gives an insight into various staff roles from the outset. As well as training, it is beneficial to gain rapport from the outset with various members of staff working in the environment, and a good way to do this is to ask to shadow a shift. This was a skill learned in an earlier study of a similar nature, undertaken in custody suites called ACCEPT (Birch et al. 2015), where staff observed a number of night shifts in order to understand the barriers staff face hands on. It also gave an opportunity to discuss with staff, the intricacies of the research, and identify small opportunities within the "regime" that the research could be slipped in.

Ethical approval

Ethical approval will need to be sought from the university itself in the first instance, then by HMPPS; either by IRAS or the excel application depending on the subject of the research, and the amount of prisons access is required to. The turnaround is very quick in comparison to NHS ethical approval, and no meeting is required to be attended; however, the questions asked are similar to that of NHS approval, and some time will need to be set aside to complete the application. An important point to note for ethical approval in a prison is that co-production is essential from day one. The first step, even prior to submitting ethical approval documents, is getting the governor on board with the research.

Security training

Regardless of the reason an individual is beginning work in a prison (nurse, researcher, prison officer, etc.), breakaway training is required. The training involves a mix of taught and practical sessions around protecting yourself inside the prison. The day ends with a practical scenario to complete in a set up threatening situation.

Breakaway training

Breakaway training is a physical training day, undertaken by any new member of staff. The training is a mix of taught, and physical activities. Various elements of self-defence are taught by experienced prison staff, and as researchers conducting interviews, useful tips about how to conduct yourself, with your own safety in mind. It is useful to note that during these training sessions, research staff are not treated any differently; the training is given the same as if the researcher is a prison officer, and the researchers' behaviour must reflect this.

Key training

To obtain access to keys when undertaking research in a prison is as one would expect, regulated. Extra security is required, fingerprints to access the key cabinets, training around the different types of keys, and training around how to carry keys is also necessary. There are locked doors and gates every couple of feet, and this can be a new experience if it is the first time working in such an environment. A good researcher will familiarise themselves with the layout of the prison, and how to handle keys, so as to work well with prison staff and work independently, in order to carry out the research efficiently.

Conditioning

Some prisons require conditioning training to be completed. This is intended to give the individual the skills to interact with prisoners in a manner that does not threaten their own personal safety. It considers issues such as clothing and talking about personal issues or family. This can be an important training element for a researcher, as conducting interviews often leads to informal conversations, where the interviewer may let their guard down.

Entrance to the prison

Rigorous security clearance has to be undertaken for any RA to work in any prison. As mentioned above, this can include a whole range of different requirements. Security clearance sets an RA up as a visitor and a pass is issued for the prison. This pass stays at the prison. Therefore, it can still be time consuming to gain entry to the prison, and any RA should be prepared for that. The gate to a prison can be busy with various visiting legal counsel, or simply a delivery. Those individuals will need to be vetted by staff adequately to gain access. Therefore, to collect a pass from the staff to enter the prison can involve a lot of waiting around.

Summary

To conduct research effectively and efficiently in the prison setting, co-production work with the prison staff, and prisoners themselves is vital, Verschuere sums this up as: "We define co-production ... rather narrowly, as the involvement of individual citizens and groups in public service delivery" (Verschuere et al. 2012, p. 1086). The concept of co-production is not a new one. As Professor Newbury-Birch wrote: "research in the criminal justice system is difficult. There are a lot of competing parts to the equation including experience and expertise, values and judgement, resources, policy context, habits and traditions, pressure groups as well as research evidence" (Newbury-Birch 2016b, p. 130); and therefore in research sites such as prisons, this involves working closely with a range of stakeholders, all the way from the prison governor, down through wing managers, prison officers and all the way through to peer prisoners, or listeners as they are sometimes known as to enable the eclectic mix of skills to be utilised effectively.

By taking a co-production approach one avoids the problem of:

> Academics and practitioners inhabiting very different worlds. Practitioners grapple with complex social and economic issues on behalf of citizens and service users. Their actions are subject to public scrutiny and their decisions are influenced by a host of factors, often including intense political pressures. By contrast, academics enjoy an unusual degree of autonomy and many have no interest in addressing "real world" problems.
>
> (Martin 2010, p. 2)

There are incentives on both sides when doing any type of co-production or public engagement work; however, the benefits and barriers must be thought about thoroughly when designing the research. By working with the prison staff, an insight into feasibility of the actual data collection is given from the outset, and plans put into place to bulletproof against any issues that may arise. Academics simply cannot understand prison regimes without this element. There is a brilliant paper discussing the 12 restorative justice projects that took place in both the UK and Australia (Sherman et al. 2015, p. 508), which discusses the intricacies of conducting research with practitioners and mentions: "Magistrates' court clerks were not so cooperative. While two small RCTs in Northumbrian Magistrates' Courts were eventually completed, their samples were only achieved by the dogged persistence of the Northumbria Manager, Dorothy Newbury-Birch", which sums up the difficulties in one sentence.

The next phase of the PRISM-A study has recently started, a pilot feasibility study named APPRAISE (A two-arm parallel group individually randomised prison pilot study of a male remand alcohol intervention for self-efficacy enhancement), moving the work forward to measure how feasible it is to carry out screening and brief interventions with male remand prisoners.

Five top tips to take forward

To conclude this chapter; five take-home top tips for conducting research with prison staff, whilst working in the prison environment would be:

- **Business as usual.** Treat the data collection in the same way you would any other environment. Yes, it is prison, and vigilance is needed. However, when interacting with participants, the situation is no different to approaching someone in A&E or a school, for example. You have to fit in as effortlessly with staff as you would in any other setting. Building rapport from the outset is key, ask about regimes, ask how they prefer you work and ask if you are unsure of anything!
- **Buddy up.** Always have a "buddy". Essential in any type of research. However, in this situation, someone who understands the prison

environment. If prison is a new environment to the researcher, there will be things witnessed that can be eye opening, being able to offload to someone is a huge help. Prison staff become used to the noise, smell and events that take place, to maintain an air of confidence, and maintain rapport, a buddy will help.

- **Communicate!** Explain to all members of prison staff who you are, what you are doing, and if it helps, which rooms you are using so someone is aware of where you are at all times. From experience, if all staff, including any drug and alcohol workers, or other type of support workers are not sure what it is the project entails, you may come across some tension; breaking this barrier from the outset can be very helpful for both parties.
- **Personal alarm**. Not all prison staff carry a personal alarm. However, they are available, and, as researchers, wearing one (they simply clip on to your belt) has no impact other than enhanced safety and an enhanced sense of confidence. Also, from experience, officers on the wing will feel more at ease if they have less to worry about in terms of safety.
- **Patience**. It can be timely to merely get through the gate. It is important to remember that this is exactly the same for all other members of prison staff, and if they can deal with it day in, day out, so can a researcher. Then there can be a number of alarms going off one after another; or a "lockdown" meaning the research will have to be put on hold until the issue is resolved. There can also be certain epidemics taking place, for example, when there are issues with new NPS such as Spice, security can tighten and every member of staff can be searched thoroughly – extending that time at the gate further. It is also worth noting, if paperwork is needed for research, such as questionnaires, these need to go through security scanners, again holding entry up. Patience really is a virtue.

References

NPC (2012.). *Safe management and use of controlled drugs in prison health in England. United Kingdom*. London: National Institute for Health and Clinical Excellence, NICE.

Babor, T., De La Fuente, J., Saunders, J. and Grant, M. (1989). *AUDIT, The Alcohol Use Disorders Identification Test, guidelines for use in primary health care*. Geneva, World Health Organisation.

Birch, J., Scott, S., Newbury-Birch, D., Brennan, A., Brown, H., Coulton, S., Gilvarry, E., Hickman, M., McColl, E., McGovern, R., Muirhead, C. and Kaner, E. (2015.). "A pilot feasibility trial of alcohol screening and brief intervention in the police custody setting (ACCEPT): study protocol for a cluster randomised controlled trial." *Pilot and Feasibility Studies* 1:6.

Coulton, S., Newbury-Birch, D., Cassidy, P., Dale, V., Deluca, P., Gilvarry, E., Godfrey, C., Heather, N., Kaner, E., Oyefeso, A., Parrott, S., Phillips, T., Shepherd, J. and Drummond, C. (2012.). "Screening for alcohol use in criminal justice settings: an exploratory study." *Alcohol Alcohol* 47(4): 423–427.

Craig, P., Dieppe, P.Macintyre, S.Michie, S.Nazareth, I.Petticrew, M. and Medical Research Council (2008). "Developing and evaluating complex interventions: the new Medical Research Council guidance." *BMJ* 337(7676): 979–983.

Fazel, S.D. and Baillargeon, J. P. (2011). "The health of prisoners." *Lancet*, 377(9769): 956–965.

Government., U. (2012.). *Health and Social Care Act (2012)*. London: Stationery Office.

Holloway, A., Landale, S., Ferguson, J., Newbury-Birch, D., Parker, R., Smith, P. and Sheikh, A. (2017). "Alcohol Brief Interventions (ABIs) for male remand prisoners: protocol for development of a complex intervention and feasibility study (PRISM-A)." *BMJ Open* 7(4): e014561.

Kok, G., Gottlieb, N.H., Peters, G.-J.Y., Mullen, P.D., Parcel, G.S., Ruiter, R.A.C., Fernández, M.E., Markham, C. and Bartholomew, L.K. (2016). "A taxonomy of behaviour change methods: an Intervention Mapping approach." *Health Psychology Review* 10(3): 297–312.

Library., H. o. C. (2018). *Briefing Paper, "UK Prison Population Statistics"*. Number CBP-04334.

Mah, D. Y., Prakash, A., Porras, D., Fynn-Thompson, F., DeWitt, E.S. and Banka, P. (2018). "Coronary artery compression from epicardial leads: More common than we think." *Heart rhythm* 15(10): 1439–1447.

Martin, S. (2010). "Co-production of social research: strategies for engaged scholarship." *Public Money & Management* 30(4): 211–218.

Newbury-Birch, D., McGovern, R., Birch, J., O'Neill, G., Kaner, H., Sondhi, A. and Lynch, K. (2016a). "A rapid systematic review of what we know about alcohol use disorders and brief interventions in the criminal justice system." *International Journal of Prisoner Health*. 12(1): 57–70.

Newbury-Birch, D., Coulton, S., Bland, M., Cassidy, P., Dale, V., Deluca, P., Gilvarry, E., Godfrey, C., Heather, N., Kaner, E., McGovern, R., Myles, J., Oyefeso, A., Parrott, S., Patton, R., Perryman, K., Phillips, T., Shepherd, J. and Drummond, C. (2014.). "Alcohol screening and brief interventions for offenders in the probation setting (SIPS Trial): A pragmatic multicentre cluster randomised controlled trial,." *Alcohol Alcohol*. 49(5): 540–554.

Newbury-Birch, D., Ferguson, J., Landale, S., Giles, E.L., McGeechan, G.J., Gill, C., Stockdale, K. and Holloway, A. (2018.). "A systematic review of the efficacy of alcohol interventions for incarcerated people." *Alcohol Alcohol* 53(4): 412–425.

Newbury-Birch, D., Harrison, B., Brown, N. and Kaner, E. (2009.). "Sloshed and sentenced: a prevalence study of alcohol use disorders amongst offenders in the North East of England. ." *International Journal of Prisoner Health*. 5(4): 201–211.

Newbury-Birch, D., McGeechan, G. and Holloway, A. (2016b). "Climbing down the steps from the ivory tower: how UK academics and practitioners need to work together on alcohol studies. Editorial." *International Journal of Prisoner Health*. 12 (3): 129–134.

Office, N.A. (2017). *A short guide to the Ministry of Justice*. M. o. Justice, NAO External Relations DP Ref.

Sherman, L.W., Strang, H., Barnes, G., Woods, D.J., Bennett, S., Inkpen, N., Newbury-Birch, D., Rossner, M., Angel, C., Mearns, M. and Slothower, M. (2015). "Twelve experiments in restorative justice: the Jerry Lee program of randomized trials of restorative justice conferences." *Journal of Experimental Criminology*. 11(4): 501–540.

Sondhi, A., Birch, J., Lynch, K., Holloway, A. and Newbury-Birch, D. (2016.). "Exploration of delivering brief interventions in a prison setting: A qualitative study in one English region." *Drugs Education, Prevention and Policy.* 23(5): 382–387.

Ministry of Justice (2018). *Offender Management Statistics Quarterly.* London: National Statistics.

Verschuere, B., Brandsen, T. and Pestoff, V. (2012). "Co-production: The state of the art in research and the future agenda." *Voluntas: International Journal of Voluntary and Nonprofit Organizations* 23(4): 1083–1101.

10 Police officers and academics working together

Dorothy Newbury-Birch, Tony Power, Angela Tomlinson, Mark Hatcher and Mick Urwin

In 1998, Lawrence Sherman advocated for "evidence-based policing", arguing that "police practices should be based on scientific evidence about what works best" (Sherman 1998). Like other police researchers and innovative police chiefs at the time, Sherman argued that rigorous and systematic scientific research should be used and generated by the police to make both tactical and strategic decisions. However, as others have argued, this information needs to be translated into everyday decision-making (Sherman 1998; Newbury-Birch et al. 2016a). This approach is now recognised as the best, and correct, way to conduct research in the police setting (Sherman et al. 1997; Farrington et al. 2002). However, practitioners often want, and, in fact, need 'quick fix' answers to complex problems and telling them that a project may take two years or longer to complete is frustrating to them (Newbury-Birch et al. 2016a). It is therefore important, some would argue, imperative, to include practitioners and individuals involved in the police service in all stages of research (Newbury-Birch et al. 2016b). By doing this, both academics and police staff can share experiences and learning with and from each other. This is summed up perfectly by Shepherd, 2014, as evidence needing to flow through the ecosystem from generation to end-user, where both push and pull are needed (Shepherd 2014).

However, when it comes to informing policy there tends to be an over reliance on evidence from university led, tightly controlled intervention trials, which can lead to questions about the applicability of research in the real world (Pettman et al. 2012). It is important that strategies be put into place that ensure that we utilise a co-production method of working with practitioners and of course service users where possible (Sherman et al. 2015; Newbury-Birch et al. 2016b). Whilst it has been argued academics and criminal justice practitioners may be seen by many as coming from two very different places, the boundaries between them may not be as large as many believe (Wehrens 2014), and a co-production approach where researchers and police working together could lead to real translational research (Graham and Tetroe 2007).

Research in the criminal justice system is difficult. There are a lot of competing parts to the equation including experience and expertise; values and judgement; resources; policy context; habits and traditions; the influence of pressure groups as well as research evidence (Armstrong et al. 2014; Newbury-Birch et al. 2014; Sherman et al. 2015; Newbury-Birch et al. 2016a; Newbury-Birch et al. 2016b) and for many these competing parts are hard to navigate, therefore showing the importance of working together.

One important thing to consider for participants is the perceived coercion and vulnerability involved in taking part in research. We need to ensure that participants enter into research of their own free will with the correct information given to them. It is thought, by some, that some may want to take part to have an influence on their case. However this has been shown not to be the case if research is carried out ethically and to protocol (Sherman et al. 2015) this is important when devising projects and submitting ethical approvals.

This chapter will focus on the intricacies of police officers and academics co-producing and carrying out research projects. It will focus on two studies:

1 **The UK Restorative Justice Study** (Strang et al. 2006; Sherman et al. 2007; Sherman et al. 2015) in police stations across England (Northumbria and the Metropolitan Police Force).
2 A pilot feasibility cluster randomised controlled trial of alcohol screening and brief intervention in the police custody setting: **The ACCEPT study** (Birch et al. 2015).

The UK Restorative Justice study

Aim of study: to carry out a series of randomised control trials in youth offending teams, magistrates courts, probation service and crown courts of the effectiveness of restorative justice in reducing recidivism compared to normal practice (Sherman et al. 2007; Sherman et al. 2015).

Restorative Justice delivery is based on a conference that is organised by a trained facilitator, who can invite anyone who is affected by a crime or its aftermath to attend. Invited participants include victims, offenders, their friends and family as well as community members where necessary; offenders agree in advance to "decline to deny" their commission of the crime, and to accept responsibility for causing harm, but a Restorative Justice Conference does not depend on a formal admission of guilt; There is no limit to how long a conference may last; 1–3 hours is typical (Sherman et al. 2015).

The Restorative Justice Conference has three phases:

1 Offenders describe what they did; others may add details.
2 All then consider who was affected by the crime and how, including offenders; this phase is often highly emotional, sometimes with shouts and tears, which gives victims a voice and offenders the chance to realise the impact of the crime.

3   The final phase is a discussion and decision about what needs to happen to repair the harm the crime caused and to ensure that it will not be repeated. This often involves the offender agreeing to perform reparation. (Sherman et al. 2015)

These can be reduced to three key questions (principles), which should be posed by the facilitator in orchestrating the discussion:

- What happened?
- Who was affected?
- What is to be done?

(Sherman et al. 2015)

In the North East of England Professor Newbury-Birch and her research assistant worked in the two police stations with the eight police officers involved in the project (including Angela Tomlinson, Tony Power and Mark Hatcher). There was a lead police officer who line managed the police officers. Professor Newbury-Birch was line managed by the one of the Chief Investigators of the study, Dr Heather Strang. Daily meetings were held between Professor Newbury-Birch and the police officers in managing the research project and participant recruitment. Decisions were made by the team but ratified by the chief police officer and the Chief Investigators of the research study: Dr Heather Strang and Professor Lawrence Sherman. This enabled those working on the project to discuss and sort out issues as they came up. Recruitment was slow in some of the studies and Sherman described the fact that they were finished was down to the "dogged persistence of Professor Newbury-Birch" (Sherman et al. 2015) and whereas this may be true, it was definitely down to the relationship built between the team and other partners.

There were, however, issues in how the research was conducted. Whereas in the other areas of the research study researchers were given access to online police data, this did not happen in the North East, which meant that the researchers were dependent on the police officers. There were sometimes issues where the lead police and chief investigators disagreed on how things should proceed, which meant that the researchers and police officers were not always sure of decision-making. Restorative justice was a new process for the police at this time point which meant that changes had to be made to how to manage work, how to record what was happening and crucially how to share data with several outside agencies. The positive outcome was that the researchers and police learned a lot about each other's roles and needs, while the downside was that this sometimes slowed progress while waiting for ratification, or obstructed progress if police or other agencies were reluctant or unwilling to share data.

The ACCEPT study

Aim of study: to investigate whether a definitive evaluation of screening and brief interventions aimed at reducing risky drinking in arrestees is acceptable and feasible in the custody suite setting (Birch et al. 2015). The project involved screening for risky drinking amongst those people who had been arrested. Detention officers (or drug and alcohol workers) were cluster randomised to one of three conditions: screening only (control group), screening followed immediately by 10 min of manualised brief structured advice delivered by the individual responsible for screening (intervention 1) or screening followed by 10 min of manualised brief structured advice delivered by the individual responsible for screening plus the offer of a subsequent 20-min session of behaviour change counselling delivered by a trained alcohol health worker (intervention 2).

There is an extensive body of evidence which demonstrates the link between risky drinking, risky behaviours and criminal activity (Newbury-Birch et al. 2009; Barton 2011; Orr et al. 2015). It has been noted that a quarter of police time is spent on dealing with alcohol-related crime (Palk et al. 2007) and the cost to the UK economy has been shown to be around £11 billion each year (Alcohol Team Home Office 2013). Therefore finding effective interventions is necessary. Alcohol screening and brief alcohol intervention is a secondary preventative approach (Kaner et al. 2008), which involves the identification via screening of risky drinking and the delivery of an intervention aimed at reducing consumption and concomitant problems. There is a wealth of evidence in primary care for the effectiveness of alcohol approach (Kaner et al. 2008; O'Donnell et al. 2014), however there has been very little research carried out in the criminal justice system, which means that this research is imperative to the evidence base (Newbury-Birch et al. 2016b).

Participants were aged 18+ who screened positive on the Alcohol Use Disorders Identification Test (Babor et al. 1989). Participants were then followed up at 6 and 12 months post-intervention. An embedded qualitative process evaluation explored acceptability of alcohol screening and brief intervention to staff and arrestees as well as facilitators and barriers to the delivery of such approaches in this setting (Birch et al. 2015).

Results showed that, of 3330 arrestees approached: 2228 were eligible for screening (67%) and 720 consented to take part in the study (32%); 386 (54%) scored 8+ on AUDIT (Babor et al. 1989); and 205 (53%) were enrolled into the study (79 controls, 65 brief advice and 61 brief counselling). Follow-up rates at 6 and 12 months were 29% and 26%, respectively. However, routinely collected re-offending data were obtained for 193 (94%) participants. Qualitative data showed that all arrestees reported awareness that participation was voluntary, that the trial was separate from police work, and the majority said trial procedures were acceptable (Addison et al. 2018).

Unlike the Restorative Justice study researchers were not based at the police station; however, they spent a lot of time there to ensure they knew the individuals involved in the study and could answer any questions. Sgt Mick Urwin was vital to how this worked. He facilitated access to the police stations and sent emails to relevant people to ensure that the project was carried out to the agreed protocol. He was involved in the decision-making for the project and regularly met with the researcher(s) on the project to discuss progress.

These two, very different methodological studies show how important it is to the research field to share experiences and work together in developing and carrying out research. More work is definitely needed in how we increase follow-up rates for research studies with this population.

Top five tips

- Clear role descriptions at the beginning of the project, which are then reviewed regularly should be set up.
- Where possible, researchers and police officers should be involved in the decision making of any project.
- Researchers, if possible, should be embedded, at least part time, with the police officers involved.
- A good working relationship between researchers and police officers should be nurtured and encouraged.
- Police officers should be briefed prior to the project commencing to understand the aims/objectives and to understand why research takes time and that it is not something that will happen overnight. Patience is required. Police officers tend to identify a problem – deal with it and move on to the next one in quick time.

References

Addison, M., R. McGovern, C. Angus, F. Becker, A. Brennan, H. Brown, S. Coulton, L. Crowe, E. Gilvarry, M. Hickman, D. Howel, E. McColl, C. Muirhead, D. Newbury-Birch, M. Waqas and E. Kaner (2018). "Alcohol screening and brief intervention police custody suites: Pilot cluster randomised controlled trial (AcCePT)." *Alcohol Alcohol*: 1–18.

Alcohol Team Home Office (2013). *Next steps following the consultation on delivering the Government's alcohol strategy.* London: Home Office.

Armstrong, R., T.L. Pettman and E. Waters (2014). "Shifting sands – from description to solutions." *Public Health* 128(6): 525–532.

Babor, T., J. De La Fuente, J. Saunders and M. Grant (1989). *AUDIT, the Alcohol Use Disorders Identification Test, guidelines for use in primary health care.* Geneva: World Health Organisation.

Barton, A. (2011). "Screening and Brief Intervention of Detainees for Alcohol use: A Social Crime Prevention Approach to Combating Alcohol-Related Crime?" *The Howard Journal* 50(1): 62–74.

Birch, J., S. Scott, D. Newbury-Birch, A. Brennan, H. Brown, S. Coulton, E. Gilvarry, M. Hickman, E. McColl, R. McGovern, C. Muirhead and E. Kaner (2015). "A pilot feasibility trial of alcohol screening and brief intervention in the police custody setting (ACCEPT): study protocol for a cluster randomised controlled trial." *Pilot and Feasibility Studies* 1(1): 6.

Farrington, D., D. MacKenzie, L. Sherman and B. Welsh (2002). *Evidence-based crime prevention*. London: Routledge.

Graham, I. D. and J. Tetroe (2007). "How to translate health research knowledge into effective healthcare action." *Healthcare Q* 10: 20–22.

Kaner, E. F. S., H. O. Dickinson, F. Beyer, E. Piennar, F. Campbell, C. Schlesinger, N. Heather, J. Saunders and B. Burnand (2008). *Effectiveness of brief alcohol interventions in primary care populations* (Review). Oxford: The Cochrane Collaboration.

Newbury-Birch, D., M. Bland, P. Cassidy, S. Coulton, P. Deluca, C. Drummond, E. Gilvarry, C. Godfrey, N. Heather, E. Kaner, J. Myles, A. Oyefeso, S. Parrott, K. Perryman, T. Phillips, D. Shenker and J. Shepherd (2009). "Screening and brief interventions for hazardous and harmful alcohol use in probation services: a cluster randomised controlled trial protocol." *BMC Public Health* 9: 418.

Newbury-Birch, D., S. Coulton, M. Bland, P. Cassidy, V. Dale, P. Deluca, E. Gilvarry, C. Godfrey, N. Heather, E. Kaner, R. McGovern, J. Myles, A. Oyefeso, S. Parrott, R. Patton, K. Perryman, T. Phillips, J. Shepherd and C. Drummond (2014). "Alcohol screening and brief interventions for offenders in the probation setting (SIPS Trial): a pragmatic multicentre cluster randomised controlled trial." *Alcohol & Alcoholism* 49(5): 540–548.

Newbury-Birch, D., G. McGeechan and A. Holloway (2016a). "Climbing down the steps from the ivory tower: How UK academics and criminal justice practitioners need to work together on alcohol studies." *International Journal of Prisoner Health* 12(3): 129–134.

Newbury-Birch, D., R. McGovern, J. Birch, G. O'Neill, H. Kaner, A. Sondhi and K. Lynch (2016b). "A rapid systematic review of what we know about alcohol use disorders and brief interventions in the criminal justice system." *International Journal of Prisoner Health* 12(1): 57–70.

O'Donnell, A., E. Kaner, D. Newbury-Birch, B. Schulte, C. Schmidt, J. Reimer and P. Anderson (2014). "The impact of brief interventions in primary healthcare: A systematic review of reviews." *Alcohol Alcohol* 49(1): 66–78.

Orr, K., A. McAuley, L. Graham and S. McCoard (2015). "Applying an Alcohol Brief Intervention (ABI) model to the community justice setting: Learning from a pilot project." *Criminology and Criminal Justice* 15(1): 83–101.

Palk, G., J. Davey and J. Freeman (2007). "Policing alcohol-related incidents: a study of time and prevalence." *Policing: An International Journal of Police Strategies and Management* 30(1): 82–92.

Pettman, T., R. Armstrong, J. Doyle, B. Burford, L. Anderson, T. Hilgrove and E. Waters (2012). "Strengthening evaluation to capture the breadth of public health practice: ideal vs real." *Journal of Public Health* 37(2): 151–155.

Shepherd, J. (2014). *How to achieve more effective services: The evidence eco-system*. Cardiff: Cardiff University.

Sherman, L. (1998). *Evidence-based policing Washington, USA*, http://www.police foundation.org/.

Sherman, L., D. Gottfredson, D. MacKenzie, J. Eck, P. Reuter and S. Bushway (1997). *Preventing crime: What works, what doesn't, what's promising: A report to the United States Congress*. College Park, MD: University of Maryland.

Sherman, L., H. Strang, G. Barnes, S. Bennett, C. Angel, D. Newbury-Birch, D. Woods and C. Gill (2007). *Restorative justice: the evidence*London: Smith Institute.

Sherman, L., H. Strang, G. Barnes, D. Woods, S. Bennett, N. Inkpen, D. Newbury-Birch, M. Rossner, C. Angel, M. Mearns and M. Slothower (2015). "Twelve experiments in restorative justice: The Jerry Lee Program of randomized trials of restorative justice conferences." *Journal of Experimental Criminology* 11: 501–540.

Strang, H., L. Sherman, C. Angel, D. Woods, S. Bennett, D. Newbury-Birch and N. Inkpen (2006). "Victim evaluations of face-to-face restorative justice conferences: A quasi-experimental analysis." *Journal of Social Issues* 62(2): 281–306.

Wehrens, R. (2014). "Beyond two communities – from research utilization and knowledge translation to coproduction?" *Public Health* 128(6): 545–551.

11 Discussion

What are the barriers and facilitators to co-production working and tools for working effectively?

Dorothy Newbury-Birch and Keith Allan

In this final chapter we will look at the barriers and facilitators described in previous sections and explore how these may be addressed. In the preceding chapters we have explored what co-production *can* mean, with a particular emphasis on co-producing work between academics and public health practitioners, and brought focus to why co-production can be valuable to these groups. We have seen that partnerships can work across a range of stakeholders including academics, public health teams, schools, public services such as police forces and members of the public.

As a delivery model for public health improvement, co-production can be seen as the sharing of information and expertise making between practitioners and career researchers or academics, which when effectively applied can provide robust evaluations, improve services, and enable all partners to become more effective agents of change (Wehrens 2014; Newbury-Birch et al. 2016).

We have seen how the resource represented by co-produced projects can be valuable to health services and local authorities and indeed the scope for adding to the evidence base, not least through translational research and practice (McGeechan 2016a; McGeechan et al. 2016b; McGeechan et al. 2016c; McGeechan et al. 2018a; McGeechan et al. 2018b; McGeechan et al. 2018c; McGeechan in press). Furthermore, it can address the often-long delays between evidence generation and translation of other models (Glasgow 2003). Co-production then can be an engine for providing an evidence base for guidelines in a timely fashion.

It has been noted that evaluation of programmes and research itself can be expensive. Through consolidating programmes under an embedded researcher and co-producing projects so that, from the practitioner point of view the context is understood, a greater efficiency can be achieved and better quality evaluations delivered at an acceptable cost. These evaluations, being of a research standard, can then be used to add to the literature. An additional operational benefit for practitioners is that this co-production model tends to promote closer ties between a research unit and practitioner team. This may, for example, allow practitioners to access facilities such as university libraries and online journal collections. In this book we have also seen how this can be a workforce development opportunity for practitioners to undertake their own research as part of their day-to-day work.

A number of recommendations have been made from the practitioner and academic points of view that promote integration of participants within a co-production work stream, common to both are the need to provide appropriate training, to agree the scope of projects at the outset, to maintain communication links, and perhaps most vitally in co-production the need to treat all stakeholders equitably and ensure that all have an equal chance to speak and be heard.

Top tips for practitioners

- **Find the right academic** – Finding the correct mix of academics and practitioners to work on the project is key. The group must often make pragmatic decisions to allow for evidence to be generated in a context usually focussed on delivery. Budgets allocated to the project may be relatively small and the embedded researcher may be relatively junior in their academic career. It is therefore useful if there is also a senior researcher overseeing the work from an academic point of view. It is therefore crucial to keep good lines of communication open between all parties. Openness and approachability are also useful key traits in this context.
- **Screen for eligible projects (ensure there is baseline data)** – The programmes / interventions put forward for evaluation must meet a set criteria to be viable. Careful consideration must be given to which projects represent the best use of the co-production resource, for example there should be confidence that data are available to analyse or that it can be generated during the life of the project. This can best be supported through early multidisciplinary meetings at which timelines for projects should be established and the available resource clearly outlined and assigned.
- **Maintain clarity of roles and responsibilities** – It is critical that, in this complex relationship, all parties know their roles and responsibilities. These should be made clear, agreed and recorded at the outset. From a practitioner point of view these can be embedded within practitioner work-plans. Timelines must also be clear to effectively project manage the collaboration. There should also be clear terms of reference agreed with a project steering group comprised of stakeholders appropriate to the project. These terms of reference should cover aspects such as how the group will ensure the voices of all parties within the group will be heard as well as agreed reporting dates. Minimum datasets to be collected can also be usefully discussed at that point.
- **Do not over commit** – There is a limit to how many co-produced projects individuals can be involved with or run. Where it is not the sole focus of a practitioner's work they may be only able to participate within a single project. The calls of working in a more academic fashion may be unfamiliar and will likely represent an increased call on available time. If

projects are to be truly co-produced there needs to be an equitable balance of time put in by both the academic and practitioner partners. Co-production projects should not be seen in the same light as simply commissioning an evaluation but as an opportunity to create a more robust and insightful project.

- **Understand political landscape and changing/emerging priorities** – There are often significant pressures on public health budgets and practitioners must make the most of public money. There may be a need to prioritise some areas or projects over others to meet local priorities and needs. The evidence created during a co-production programme may be useful in making the case in setting priorities in an evidence based fashion. If working on a project that has the potential to have widespread impact there may be a need to quickly adapt to new priorities. This can be facilitated by having a good understanding of available resource and the ability to move it from one project to another, particularly if one has slack time or can be deprioritised. For this reason there needs to be good project management of all co-production projects.
- **Contributing to the evidence base** – The work undertaken will result in poster and oral presentations, as well as publications. This can be used to raise the profile of the co-production evaluation programme within the practitioner environment and demonstrate the added value of relatively small scale evaluations being conducted in the context of public health teams which is of relevance to local level priorities.

Top tips from the academic perspective

- **Co-production benefits both academics and practitioners, and can result in valuable shared learning** – There may, however, be circumstances where the academic findings do not chime with the practitioner's experience of a service or indeed fit the wider political view, this may be initially difficult but lead to greater insights useful to creating more efficient interventions or policies. There is a benefit to be had in collaborating on study questions and hypotheses; by exploring with partners primary outcomes of interest to the group new ideas may be expressed and researchers should be more likely to see their research put into practice.
- **Pressure points can cause conflict, but can be overcome through well-discussed and thought-through projects** – Academics should be aware of the competing pressures of funding priorities, teaching commitments and other duties. These will be set against the practitioner's priorities of providing a cost effective service, possibly against a politically charged background. Differences between expected practitioner evaluation and researcher timelines, again with outside pressures such as the need to commission within a cycle are also potential pressure points. Practitioners may require rapid answers to specific questions of evaluation, and a timeline of several years to provide a fully robust study may not be

acceptable. It is therefore necessary for academic partners to collaborate with their practitioner partners as fully as possible through each stage of the programme, including its planning. It may be that process or interim measures may meet the immediate needs of the practitioner with longer term outcomes being available later for more scientific study.

- **Co-produced research should benefit multiple stakeholders** – The above points can be addressed through maintaining a strong shared focus on improving population health and creating stronger communities. Effective communication is the lynch pin of this and is required between all stakeholders. In this way expectations and needs can be expressed and managed from the beginning. There is a clear need to carefully communicate the nature of the benefit which may be realised. For example, in the case of work co-produced within the justice system it should be made clear that participation in research will not affect sentencing and similarly within the health service participation will not affect social or medical care. This is part of the required informed consenting process but should be maintained throughout the project to avoid participants feeling coerced.
- **Embedding researchers in public health teams and practitioners in academic units is highly beneficial** – Here honorary contracts allow members of the different groups to embed within collaborating organisations. This can allow better access to people and data but also serves to give context and allow the embedded person to better understand the culture of the host organisations and foster useful professional networks. It is also of paramount importance that researchers gain the correct accreditation to work either in their embedded site or within the institution they are drawing their primary data from.

In conclusion, there are both limitations and strengths to the co-production model as described in this book. There are of course tensions that may be ameliorated through careful planning of projects and management of expectation. An academic may be focussed on developing research for publication within peer viewed journals. Practitioners may be more concerned with pragmatically putting available evidence into action. Another major source of potential disruption is around timelines. Both academics and practitioners noted that it was a significant factor for them to overcome during co-production projects. This can be in terms of set-up time and the need to go through ethics committees, a process largely unfamiliar to practitioners, and the differences in time a practitioner is expected to report and take action in compared with the time necessary to bring a peer reviewed journal article to publication. Furthermore, there is the tension between the robustness of the research and how quickly it can be done.

The importance of co-production research therefore lies in the sharing of skills, knowledge, and experience of both the researcher and practitioner. There are far more strengths than limitations when employing a co-production model. There is a chance to share expertise and acquire new skills. The key question is, "how do we make a positive difference?" and this leads to a true strength of co-production; it allows research to move from pure theory into directly influencing policy and practice in a direct way. As has been previously discussed interventions may be created using established academic theories yet fail to have the degree of impact expected. This may be because the individual context in which it is to be implemented is not fully understood and they are therefore a poor fit for the local environment. Co-production as a process will address this by allowing for the input of a wider range of partners. This should serve to make any intervention more locally appropriate and also increase its value in the eyes of those asked to deliver and participate in it. This in turn is likely to make a given intervention more successful and increase its longevity.

The co-production approach is especially useful for complex public health issues that have a range of drivers and potential actors upon them. They allow response to be built that goes beyond siloed working and promote engagement whilst fostering the creation of networks. This of course needs senior leadership buy in and support of this change in approach.

Embedding researchers within the host organisation be it a prison, school, local authority, third sector body or community can help enrich the project by allowing for communication of culture, they may also act as "a pair of fresh eyes"(Newbury-Birch et al. 2016). Furthermore, we know that having agency in one's own life increases the chances of a person being healthy and increases wellbeing. Therefore their inclusion in the evidence generating process will have a salutogenic effect.

The prospect of embedded researchers or co-production can be daunting for some partners. There can be a feeling of having an outsider within the camp and an anxiety at what they might discover or what their perceptions of existing structures may be. There should be awareness on all sides that partners are opening themselves to scrutiny and exposing potential vulnerabilities. The relationships must therefore be handled sensitively with briefs understood and agreed, whilst not shying away from expressing truths found. A high degree of trust between partners is therefore needed and a culture of openness and honesty maintained. Through this approach partners become colleagues rather than external agents. Again the importance of clear communication is key, as is the ability to deal with emergent change. While objectives should be agreed early it may be helpful to display understanding and flexibility in how those are best met.

Co-production, as a mutualistic project, empowers all partners involved and provides for a range of views and information to be brought together to address complex issues. It can be used to foster agency over issues that affect the lives of those involved in the research, thereby narrowing inequities and providing lasting positive change.

References

Glasgow, R. E., E. Lichtenstein and A. C. Marcus (2003). "Why don't we see more translation of health promotion research to practice?" *Am J Public Health* 93(8): 1261–1267.

McGeechan, G., K. Wilkinson, N. Martin, L. Wilson, G. O'Neill and D. Newbury-Birch (2016a). "A mixed method outcome evaluation of a specialist Alcohol Hospital Liaison Team." *Perspectives in Public Health* 136(6), 361–367.

McGeechan, G., D. Woodhall, L. Anderson, L. Wilson, G. O'Neill and D. Newbury-Birch (2016c). "A coproduction community based approach to reducing smoking prevalence in a local community setting." *Journal of Environmental and Public Health*: 538653.

McGeechan, G. R., L. Wilson, G. O'Neill, and D. Newbury-Birch (2016b). "Exploring men's perceptions of a community based men's shed programme in England." *Journal of Public Health* 39(4):e251–e256.

McGeechanm, G. J., B. M., K. Allan, G. O'Neill and D. Newbury-Birch (2018a). "Exploring young women's perspectives of a targeted support programme for teenage parents." *BMJ Sexual & Reproductive Health* 44(4): 272–277.

McGeechan, G., D. Phillips, L. Wilson, V. J. Whittaker, G. O'Neill and D. Newbury-Birch, (2018b). "Service evaluation of an exercise on referral scheme for adults with existing health conditions in the United Kingdom." *International J Behav Med* 25: 304–311.

McGeechan, G. J., C. Richardson, K. Weir, L. Wilson, G. O'Neill and D. Newbury-Birch, (2018c). "Evaluation of a police led suicide early alert surveillance strategy in the United Kingdom." *Injury Prevention* 24: 267–271.

McGeechan, G. J., C. Richardson, L. Wilson, K. Allan and D. Newbury-Birch (in press). "A qualitative exploration of a school based mindfulness course for young people." *Child and Adolescent Mental Health*.

Newbury-Birch, D., G. McGeechan and A. Holloway (2016). "Climbing down the steps from the ivory tower: how UK academics and criminal justice practitioners need to work together on alcohol studies." *International Journal of Prisoner Health* 12(3): 129–134.

Wehrens, R. (2014). "Beyond two communities – from research utilization and knowledge translation to coproduction?" *Public Health* 128(6): 545–551.

Index

Note: bold page numbers indicate tables.